Screening for Hearing Loss and Otitis Media in Children

WITHDRAWN

Screening for Hearing Loss and Otitis Media in Children

Edited by

Jackson Roush, Ph.D.

Professor and Director
Division of Speech and Hearing Sciences
The University of North Carolina School of Medicine
Chapel Hill, North Carolina

SINGULAR
™
THOMSON LEARNING

Australia   Canada   Mexico   Singapore   Spain   United Kingdom   United States

MW

SINGULAR
★
™
THOMSON LEARNING

Screening for Hearing Loss and Otitis Media in Children

Edited by

Jackson Roush, Ph.D

Business Unit Director:
William Brottmiller

Acquisitions Editor:
Marie Linvill

Developmental Editor:
Kristin Banach

COPYRIGHT © 2001 by Singular,
an imprint of Delmar, a division of
Thomson Learning, Inc.
Thomson Learning™ is a trademark
used herein under license

Printed in Canada
1 2 3 4 5 XXX 06 05 04 02 01

For more information contact
Singular,
401 West "A" Street, Suite 325
San Diego, CA 92101–7904.
Or find us on the World Wide Web
at http://www.singpub.com

Executive Marketing Manager:
Dawn Gerrain

Channel Manager:
Kathryn Little

Executive Production Editor:
Barbara Bullock

Production Editor:
Brad Bielawski

Library of Congress
Cataloging-in-Publication Data
Jackson Roush
Screening for Hearing Loss and
Otitis Media in Children/[edited by]
Jackson Roush
p.; cm

Includes bibliographic references
and index
ISBN 0-7693-0000-6
(pbk.: ALK paper)
1. Deafness in children 2. Otitis
Media in children 3. Hearing Loss,
Functional—Child 4. Hearing Loss,
Functional—Infant 5. Hearing
Tests—Methods.
WV232 5433 2001

RF291.5.C45 S374 2001
618.92'0978-dc 21 00-049254

NOTICE TO THE READER

11/21/02

Contents

Part III: Referral, Follow-Up, and Parent-Professional Communication

Foreword

Textbooks on hearing assessment focus on diagnostic methods that utilize sophisticated technology combined with the skill of the audiologist to obtain a full assessment of auditory processing, from the passive response of the external ear to the complex neural processing of the auditory cortex. These methods are so advanced that current research is largely concerned with improving already excellent tests. The greatest weakness of diagnostic audiology is that children and adults with hearing loss are not tested when they *need* to be tested. This weakness is especially egregious in view of recent compelling evidence that many lifelong sequelae of hearing loss are preventable by early identification and intervention.

Screening for Hearing Loss and Otitis Media in Children is an important resource that will help establish programs for early identification of hearing loss and middle ear disease. It is aimed at a large audience—professionals from various disciplines involved in the implementation of a screening program, in a variety of venues from the newborn nursery, to school-based screening programs, to the physician's office. While emphasizing the essential role of the audiologist, it provides sufficient basic information for the non-audiologist to understand the principles and methods, and it includes important guidelines for audiologists to select and evaluate testing protocols. It gathers together under a single cover the collective expertise of those who are most experienced in designing, implementing, and evaluating screening programs and it covers all the steps from design to implementation to referral and follow-up. Both hospital-based and school-based programs are described and guidelines are provided for the use of specific screening instruments, including auditory brainstem response, otoacoustic emissions, tympanometry, and pure tone screening.

The next great advance in the diagnosis and management of hearing disorders will not be a "super test" like Dr. McCoy's Star Trek scanner. It will be in making our current tests accessible to all children. Without one more data point on the sensitivity and specificity of current or future tests, we have the tools to significantly reduce the impact of hearing loss in our society. By following the principles and methods presented in this book, the health and welfare of many children will be improved through early identification and treatment of hearing loss and middle ear disease.

Robert H. Margolis
University of Minnesota

Preface

Hearing loss is often described as an invisible condition. Because it offers no obvious indications, undetected hearing loss in a child may be mistaken for a developmental delay or an attention deficit disorder. Furthermore, hearing loss may result in delayed speech and language development as well as impaired academic achievement or socialization. Otitis media, which is most prevalent in the early years, can also affect a child's health and development. Unlike acute episodes of middle ear disease, which are readily apparent from pain and other overt symptoms, non-infected middle ear fluid and accompanying hearing loss are often overlooked without appropriate screening procedures.

This book is intended to serve as a practical guide for professionals who encounter infants and young children in need of screening for hearing loss and otitis media: nurses, speech-language pathologists, pediatricians, and other healthcare personnel. It will also serve as a useful resource for students in these disciplines and for audiologists with limited experience in pediatric screening. Experienced audiologists will be interested in the program models described in chapters 4–9.

Throughout the text, emphasis is given to the importance of communication among professionals and with family members. Especially critical are the issues of referral and follow-up. The best intentions are of little value without careful consideration to these critical elements. In fact, a poorly designed or improperly executed screening program is likely to do more harm than good.

A successful screening program requires careful attention to numerous technical issues pertaining to methodology and instrumentation. Equally important are the interpersonal aspects: effective communication with screening personnel and referral agencies. Finally, the administrative and business aspects of the program must be fully considered. Cost analysis, reimbursement, regulatory issues, and program evaluation are essential ongoing activities.

Optimal hearing and ear health are critical to the development of young children. With careful planning, both can be accomplished in a timely and cost-effective manner. This book will have achieved its intended purpose if it serves as a useful introduction to the essential components of a screening program and as a resource for those engaged in developing or improving existing programs.

Readers' comments and suggestions can be sent, via E-mail, to jroush@med.unc.edu.

Jackson Roush
Chapel Hill, NC

Acknowledgments

Sincere thanks and appreciation go to each of the chapter contributors for sharing their clinical experience and expertise. I am also indebted to several colleagues who provided advice and editorial suggestions regarding the background information in Part I: John Grose, Judy Gravel, Barb Herrmann, Irva Hertz-Picciotto, Bob Margolis, Judith Marlowe, Bob Nozza, and Anne Marie Tharpe. Thanks also to Anne Lauder, Emily Zanzot, and Paul Braly for the preparation of figures and illustrations and to Turner McCollom for the cover design. I could not have completed this book without the capable assistance of the editors and staff of Singular-Thomson Learning: Jeff Danhauer, Candace Janco, Kristin Banach, and Brad Bielawski. I am also grateful to several graduate students at UNC Chapel Hill for helpful reviews and commentary: Amanda Panning, MaryAnne Gobble, and Keely Boyle. Finally, special thanks to my wife and colleague, Pat Roush, for her willing advice and enduring tolerance.

Jackson Roush
Chapel Hill, NC

Dedication

To Pat, Liz, Ben, and Jenny

Contributors

Janie Chobot, M.A.
Supervisor of Audiology
Children's Evaluation and Rehabilition Center
Rose F. Kennedy Center University Affiliated Program
Albert Einstein College of Medicine
Bronx, New York

Elizabeth R. Crais, Ph.D.
Professor of Speech-Language Pathology
Division of Speech and Hearing Sciences
University of North Carolina
Chapel Hill, North Carolina

Wendy G. Crumley, M.S.
Site Manager
Sounds of Texas State Project on Newborn Hearing Screening
Fort Worth, Texas

Terese Finitzo, Ph.D.
Director, Sounds of Texas State Project on Newborn Hearing Screening
Fort Worth, Texas

Judith Gravel, Ph.D
Professor of Otorhinolaryngology
Associate Professor of Pediatrics
Albert Einstein College of Medicine
Kennedy Center
Bronx, New York

Deborah Hayes, Ph.D.
Chair, Audiology, Speech Pathology, and Learning Services
The Children's Hospital
Denver, Colorado

Barbara S. Herrmann, Ph.D.
Audiologist
Department of Otology and Laryngology
Harvard Medical School
Massachusetts Eye & Ear Infirmary
Boston, Massachusetts

Mary Jane Johnson
Coordinator: The Family Guidance Early Intervention Program
Rhode Island School for the Deaf
Providence, Rhode Island

Ellen Kurtzer-White, M.S.
Project Director
First Connections Resource and Training Project
for Newborn Hearing Screening
Providence, Rhode Island

Christine Liskow, M.A.
Clinical Audiologist
Lenox Hill Hospital
Cochlear Implant Center
New York, New York

Martha Mundy, Au.D.
Clinical Instructor
Division of Speech and Hearing Sciences
University of North Carolina
Chapel Hill, North Carolina

Jackson Roush, Ph.D.
Professor and Director
Division of Speech and Hearing Sciences
University of North Carolina
Chapel Hill, North Carolina

Lisa M. Stellwagen, M.D.
Director of Newborn Nursery
Department of Pediatrics
University of California, San Diego
San Diego, California

Vickie Thomson, M.A.
State Audiology Consultant
Colorado Department of Public Health and Environment
Health Care Program for Children with Special Needs
Denver, Colorado

Aaron Thornton, Ph.D.
Associate Professor
Department of Otology and Laryngology
Harvard Medical School
Massachusetts Eye & Ear Infirmary
Boston, Massachusetts

Part I:
Preliminary Considerations

INTRODUCTION

Chapters 1 and 2 of this text provide an overview of hearing, hearing loss, principles of screening, and methodology for identification of hearing loss and otitis media with various populations. For improved readability and flow of text, terms used in Chapters 1 and 2 that may be new to some readers are italicized and defined more thoroughly in the Glossary. Chapter 3 examines developmental milestones useful in determining whether children should be referred for further evaluation.

Screening for Hearing Loss and Otitis Media: Basic Principles

Jackson Roush

INTRODUCTION

Timely identification and intervention for hearing loss has been a significant and long-standing problem in the United States and in other nations. For decades, the average age of identification for hearing loss was between two and three years, far later than it should be according to the Joint Committee on Infant Hearing (JCIH, 2000), which recommends that hearing loss at birth be identified by three months of age and intervention begun by six months of age. This goal seemed unattainable for many years but new technologies and automation of established procedures are making early identification and intervention a reality. Hospitals throughout the nation are now actively engaged in universal hearing screening, and in most states, newborn hearing screening is now required by law. Moreover, there is growing evidence that early identification followed by early intervention results in better long-term developmental outcomes for children and their families.

There is also a growing awareness of the need to detect hearing loss in older children. In regions where universal hearing screening is not available, a permanent congenital hearing loss may escape detection for months or even years. It is also possible for a permanent hearing loss to have its onset later in childhood. Finally, hearing loss caused by otitis media, although rarely permanent, can occur throughout early childhood, resulting in medical complications as well as adverse effects on communication. In some cases, delays in speech, language, or learning may ensue. Whatever the cause, undetected hearing loss or middle ear disease in children is a serious matter. Not only is appropriate intervention denied, undetected hearing loss may be mistaken for a developmental disorder or attention deficit.

It is not surprising that there are differences of opinion regarding the selection of screening methods, target populations, and who should be responsible for payment. Even so, the importance of timely identification, referral, and follow-up is widely recognized. It is also agreed that successful outcomes can only be achieved with appropriate and cost-effective protocols combined with well-qualified screening personnel. In fact, the results of a recent federally funded, multi-center research project found that skill and competence of screening personnel were critical factors in the success of a newborn hearing screening program.

This book is intended to serve as a practical guide to the design and implementation of specific protocols for the identification of hearing loss and otitis media in children. Procedures of choice differ according to the child's age and developmental status, but the goal is the same: to identify children most likely to have a hearing or middle ear disorder needing medical, audiologic, or speech-language intervention. The information in this text will be useful to professionals in a variety of settings who encounter infants and young children in need of screening for hearing loss and otitis media: audiologists, nurses, pediatricians, speech-language pathologists, and support personnel. Audiologists and otolaryngologists are responsible for the diagnosis of hearing loss, but professionals from other disciplines play a critical role in the identification and referral process. Their role in screening for hearing loss and otitis media is endorsed by both the *American Academy of Audiology* (AAA) and the *American Speech-Language-Hearing Association* (ASHA). Of course, both organizations emphasize that screening personnel must be knowledgeable, well-trained, and fully aware of their professional scope of practice. Institutional screening programs, such as those in hospital nurseries, preschools, and public schools, should be conducted under the general supervision of an audiologist. Where hearing screenings are performed on an individual basis (e.g., in a pediatrician's office) audiologic supervision is rarely available. In those settings it is especially critical for hearing and middle ear screening to be conducted accurately using appropriate methods and properly calibrated instrumentation. With the necessary knowledge and skill, a diverse array of health care providers can participate in the identification of hearing loss and otitis media in children.

Each pediatric population presents unique demands for screening personnel. For example, hearing screening in a typical school-age population, while necessitating careful planning and implementation, requires minimal equipment and preparation of screening personnel. In contrast, screening for hearing loss in a hospital neonatal intensive care unit requires special instrumentation and test procedures carefully monitored by an audiologist. Regardless of population or setting, it is imperative that screening personnel be fully qualified, and have access to the technical support needed for proper equipment selection, maintenance, and calibration. Equally important is the selection of protocols for screening and procedures for referral, follow-up, and program evaluation. State licensure laws must be carefully reviewed to ensure that hearing and middle ear screening activities are conducted in accordance with legal and institutional requirements. Similarly, guidelines and institutional policies for infection control and universal precautions should be reviewed and strictly enforced. In some settings it may be necessary to obtain parental permission prior to conducting hearing or middle ear screening. In other settings informed consent will be part of a larger institutional enrollment process. Finally, screening personnel must recognize at all times the importance of strict confidentiality regarding screening outcomes and follow-up. The procedures described in this text are consistent with the guidelines and position statements of the AAA (1997) and the ASHA (1997).

THE EAR AND HEARING

The ear transforms sound waves into nerve impulses that are transmitted to the brain. The peripheral mechanism consists of the outer, middle, and inner ear (See Figures 1–1 and 1–2). The outer ear, which includes the *pinna* and *exter-*

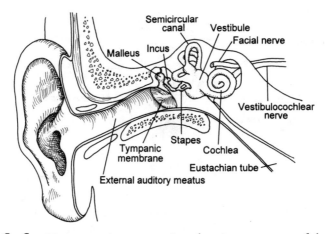

Figure 1-1 Diagrammatic cross-section showing structures of the outer, middle, and inner ear. (From *Anatomy and physiology for speech, language, and hearing, Second Ed.* (p. 566), by J. A. Seikel, D. W. King, and D. G. Drumright, 2000, San Diego, CA: Singular Publishing Group. Copyright 2000. Reprinted with permission.)

nal auditory meatus (ear canal), collects incoming sound waves and directs them to the *tympanic membrane* (eardrum). The external auditory meatus is 15–20 mm long at birth and eventually reaches an average length of 25–30 mm in adults. It is curved and progressively narrows to offer protection from trauma and foreign objects. At its medial end, the tympanic membrane forms a boundary between the outer and middle ear. It has both a tense portion or *pars tensa* as well as a smaller, more flaccid portion known as *pars flaccida* (see Figure 1–3). When sound waves enter the external meatus, the tympanic membrane moves in response to incoming sound waves and transmits the vibratory

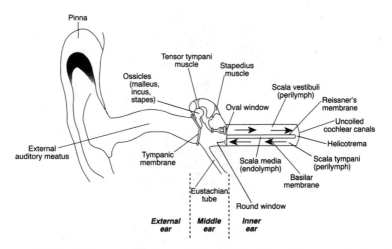

Figure 1-2 Schematic diagram of the peripheral auditory mechanism (outer, middle, and inner ear). The cochlea is "unrolled" to illustrate movement of cochlear fluids. (From *Neuroscience for the study of communicative disorders*, (p. 168), by S. C. Bhatnager and O. J. Andy, 1995, Baltimore, MD: Williams & Wilkins. Copyright 1995. Reprinted with permission.)

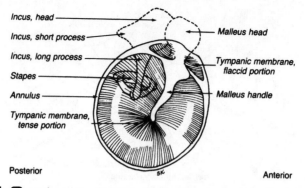

Figure 1-3 Schematic diagram of a right tympanic membrane as viewed through the otoscope. (From *Essentials of otolaryngology* (p. 7), by F. Lucente and S. Sobol, 1988, Baltimore, MD: Williams & Wilkins. Copyright 1988. Reprinted with permission.)

patterns to the middle ear, a mucous-lined and air-filled space containing a mechanical system composed of three bones, or *ossicles*: the *malleus, incus,* and *stapes* (Figure 1–4). Collectively, the ossicles transmit the mechanical energy of sound from the tympanic membrane to the fluid-filled inner ear via the oval window (see Figure 1–1). The *Eustachian tube* provides a passageway from the middle ear cavity to the throat (*nasopharynx*), where muscular contractions cause the tube to open, resulting in airflow and equalization of air pressure on either side of the tympanic membrane. Thus, the middle ear provides both air pressure equalization and a mechanical bridge between air, the source of the incoming sound energy, and fluid, which occupies the inner ear. In addition, the middle ear provides a mechanism to reduce the sound energy transmitted when

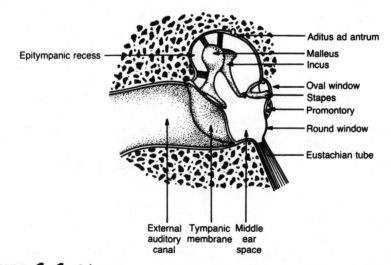

Figure 1-4 Schematic cross-section of the middle ear showing the three ossicles, *maleus, incus,* and *stapes,* which comprise the ossicular chain. (From *Introduction to audiology, Fourth Ed.* (p. 234), by F. N. Martin, 1991, Boston MA: Allyn & Bacon. Copyright 1991. Reprinted with permission.)

the ear is exposed to a loud sound. The *acoustic reflex* occurs when the *stapedius muscle* contracts in response to loud sounds, thereby stiffening the *ossicular chain* (see Figure 1–2).

The inner ear is a closed cavity containing the *membranous labyrinth*, which is encased in a *bony labyrinth* or *otic capsule*. The snail-shaped *cochlea* is composed of three ducts: the *scala vestibuli* and *scala tympani*, which contain *perilymph*, and an interior duct called the *scala media*, which contains *endolymph* (Figure 1–5). The scala media is separated from the scala vestibuli by *Reissner's membrane* and from the scala tympani by the *basilar membrane*, an elastic partition that is narrow at its base (nearest the oval window) and wide at its apex. The basilar membrane is the supporting structure for the sensory organ of hearing, the *organ of Corti*. The organ of Corti contains one row of approximately 3500 inner *hair cells* and three rows of outer hair cells, each with approximately 4000 hair cells. Projecting from the top of each hair cell are *stereocilia*, some of which are embedded in a flat overhanging mantle known as the *tectorial membrane*. As the stapes moves in and out of the oval window in response to incoming sound waves, movement of the basilar membrane causes bending

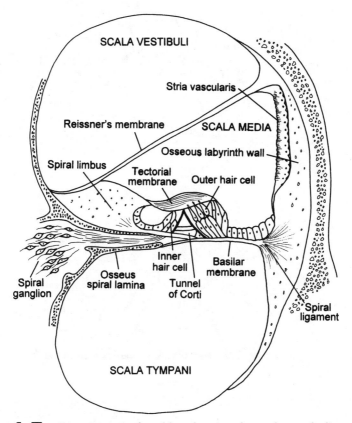

Figure 1-5 Cross-section of cochlea showing the scala vestibuli, scala media, and scala tympani. (From *Anatomy and physiology for speech, language, and hearing, Second Ed.* (p. 584), by J. A. Seikel, D. W. King, and D. G. Drumright, 2000, San Diego, CA: Singular Publishing Group. Copyright 2000. Reprinted with permission.)

of the stereocilia (Figure 1–6), which results in sensory stimulation of the hair cells, each of which is associated with a specific frequency region. As shown in Figure 1–7, the point of maximum basilar membrane displacement for low frequencies occurs at the apex, near the *helicotrema*, whereas peak displacement for high frequencies occurs at the basal end, near the oval window. Although each frequency is represented at some point along the basilar membrane, most incoming sounds have waveforms consisting of many different frequencies. Thus, movements of the basilar membrane are complex and rapidly changing. As the basilar membrane is displaced, the nerve fibers in the auditory nerve (VIIIth cranial nerve) are stimulated and, in turn, convey neural information to higher levels of the auditory system and eventually to the auditory cortex. It is important to note that the amplitude of basilar membrane displacement is determined by both the inherent mechanical (passive) properties of the membrane and by an active mechanism associated with the outer hair cells. The active mechanism reflects the "motility" of the outer hair cells, whose length varies on

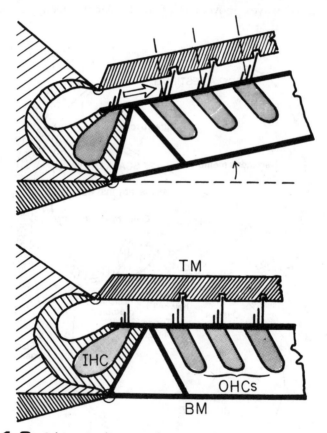

Figure 1–6 Schematic diagram of outer and inner hair cells illustrating how shearing of the stereocilia occurs as a result of basilar membrane displacement; TM = tympanic membrane, IHC = inner hair cells, OHC = outer hair cells, BM = basilar membrane (From "Physiology of the Cochlea," by A. Ryan and P. Dallos, In *Hearing Disorders, Second Ed.* (pp. 253–266), by J. L. Northern, Ed., 1984, Boston, MA: Allyn & Bacon. Copyright 1984. Reprinted with permission.)

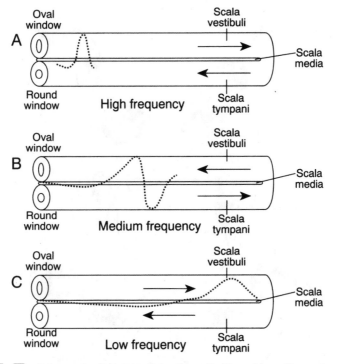

Figure 1-7 Schematic diagram of the "unrolled" cochlea, illustrating the traveling wave patterns of low, medium, and high-frequency sounds and corresponding displacements of the basilar membrane. (Adapted from *Neuroscience for the study of communicative disorders* (p. 171), by S. C. Bhatnager and O. J. Andy, 1995, Baltimore, MD: Williams & Wilkins. Copyright 1995. Reprinted with permission.)

a moment-by-moment basis in accordance with their electrochemical condition. The outer hair cells, in effect, act as cochlear amplifiers for low-level signals, a product of which is the generation of "otoacoustic emissions," described in Chapter 2. Although there are many more outer hair cells than inner hair cells, the fibers of the outer hair cells comprise only about 5% of the auditory nerve. Thus, approximately 95% of the auditory nerve fibers arise from the single row of inner hair cells. Both outer and inner hair cells and their corresponding neural elements play a critical role in hearing. The inner hair cells are associated with ascending neural fibers responsible for transmitting stimulation to higher auditory centers, while the outer hair cells respond to a descending neural feedback loop that enables the inner ear to regulate its response to incoming sounds.

In summary, air pressure waves entering the outer ear are converted to mechanical energy by the tympanic membrane and middle ear structures. The vibratory patterns are transmitted to the inner ear where they stimulate the cochlea and are transformed into nerve impulses. Taken together, the outer, middle, and inner ear comprise the *air conduction pathway*. Sound energy is also transmitted through the adjacent bone and tissue, bypassing the middle ear system and stimulating the inner ear directly via *bone conduction*. Collectively these structures comprise the peripheral auditory mechanism.

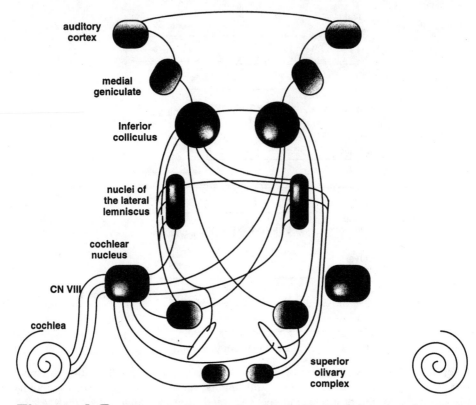

Figure 1-8 Schematic diagrams showing the major pathways and synapses of the central auditory nervous system. (From *Clinical audiology, an introduction* (p. 68), by B. A. Stach, 1998, San Diego, CA: Singular Publishing Group. Copyright 1998. Reprinted with permission. Adapted from "Structure and Function of the Central Auditory System" by G. Thompson, 1983, *Seminars in Hearing, 4 (2),* p. 9.

From the inner ear, the cochlear portion of the auditory nerve (VIIIth cranial nerve) exits the modiolus and terminates at the lower brainstem (see Figure 1–8). From the first synapse at the cochlear nucleus, most of the fibers cross to the opposite (contralateral) side of the brainstem while about one-quarter of the fibers remain on the same (ipsilateral) side. Some of the ascending fibers terminate in the lower brainstem while others extend to higher auditory centers. As shown in Figure 1–8, the major nuclei of the central auditory system include the cochlear nucleus, the lateral lemniscus, the inferior colliculus, and the medial geniculate. At the highest levels of the auditory system, fibers radiate from the medial geniculate to the auditory cortex. It is here in the brain's temporal lobe where hearing, in the perceptual sense, actually occurs.

EAR AND HEARING DISORDERS

Disorders of the External Ear

The outer ear includes the pinna and ear canal. The most common disorder of the outer ear, impacted cerumen, is also the easiest to treat. *Cerumen* (earwax) is the soft, sticky substance secreted in the ear canal. Its presence is normal and, in fact, beneficial. But excessive production of cerumen or frequent "cleaning" with a cotton swab or other implement may cause the ear canal to become occluded. Cerumen removal can usually be accomplished easily by a nurse, audiologist, or general practice physician; however, deeply impacted or hardened cerumen may require the services of an *otolaryngologist*. Other external ear disorders include *acute otitis externa* (bacterial or fungal infection) and congenital anomalies as described in Table 1–1.

Disorders of the Middle Ear

Otitis media, or inflammation of the middle ear, is highly prevalent in young children, especially during the first two years of life. In fact, otitis media is the most frequent diagnosis made by pediatricians of children under 15 years of age. Moreover, the proportion of office visits associated with otitis media has increased dramatically in recent years. Nearly 50% of all children will have at least one episode of otitis media in the first year of life and 10–20% will experience recurrent episodes during early childhood.

Although otitis media has been classified in many ways, there are basically two forms. *Acute otitis media* usually presents with sudden onset, the result of viral or bacterial agents invading the middle ear tissues and causing otalgia (pain), fever, and general discomfort. Acute otitis media often occurs during upper respiratory tract infections. Examination typically reveals a red, bulging tympanic membrane caused by purulent material in the middle ear space. Since it is difficult to determine whether the infection is viral or bacterial in nature, antibiotics are often prescribed.

The second form is *serous otitis media* or *otitis media with effusion (OME)*. This form of otitis media involves secretion of fluid from the mucous membrane lining of the middle ear. In contrast to acute otitis media, OME is generally characterized by non-infected (serous) effusion drawn into the middle ear cavity as a result of poor Eustachian tube function. Thus, OME is defined as inflammation of the middle ear with fluid present, but without obvious signs of ear infection.

TABLE 1-1 Diseases and conditions of the external ear and their treatment.	
Disease or Condition	**Description and Treatment**
Impacted Cerumen	Cerumen ("earwax"): the soft sticky substance secreted in the ear canal for the purpose of filtering debris and contaminants. Cleaning of the ear canal is necessary only if the canal becomes fully occluded.
External Otitis	Infectious or non-infectious conditions resulting in inflammation of the ear canal, which may be accompanied by pain, swelling, and discharge (otorrhea). Especially common during the summer months in the form of "swimmer's ear." Treatment usually consists of topical antibiotics.
Malformations	A variety of congenital conditions that may occur as a result of incomplete embryological development, ranging from subtle abnormalities to complete absence of the external ear. Surgical intervention is provided only if the malformations result in problems related to function or appearance.

Table 1–2 provides a summary of the various types of otitis media. Risk factors associated with the disease are summarized in Table 1–3.

Historically, the treatment of OME has varied widely among physicians. In an effort to summarize scientific evidence and develop guidelines for management of OME, the U.S. Department of Health and Human Services, through the

TABLE 1-2 Common diseases of the middle ear and their treatment.

Disease	Description and Treatment
Acute Purulent Otitis Media (AOM); also known as acute suppurative otitis media	Infection of the middle ear caused by bacterial or viral agents. Symptoms include pain and fever; characterized by sudden onset and short duration. Usually treated with antibiotics.
Otitis Media with Effusion (OME); also known as serous otitis media or secretory otitis media	Thin, watery or mucoid effusion, usually without infection and, therefore, asymptomatic other than conductive hearing loss. Most cases resolve in less than 12 weeks without treatment. When the condition is chronic or recurrent and accompanied by hearing loss, ventilation (tympanostomy) tubes are recommended.
Chronic Suppurative Otitis Media	Chronic otorrhea (drainage) through a tympanic membrane perforation. Treatment may involve topical or oral antibiotics; in some cases surgical intervention is needed to repair the perforation

TABLE 1-3 Factors associated with increased risk of otitis media (AOM and OME).

Risk Factor	Effects on Prevalence of Otitis Media
Age	Prevalence highest during infancy and early childhood.
Gender	Prevalence slightly higher in males.
Immune status	Immature immune status is associated with higher prevalence.
Other diseases and conditions	Higher prevalence associated with: • Respiratory diseases • Nasopharyngeal and upper respiratory tract infections • Adenoid or tonsillar hypertrophy • Sinusitis • Craniofacial anomalies (Down syndrome, cleft palate).
Familial clustering	Sibling and parent history are associated with higher prevalence.
Feeding practices	Breastfeeding reduces risk by providing a protective effect; supine (reclined) feeding position may lead to middle ear reflux and higher prevalence.
Child care setting	Children in group child care have higher prevalence than children in home care.
Passive smoking	Exposure to cigarette smoke is associated with higher prevalence.
Season	Prevalence is highest during the winter months.

Agency for Health Care Policy and Research (AHCPR), sponsored the development of clinical practice guidelines in a publication entitled *Otitis Media with Effusion in Young Children*. A companion document for clinicians, entitled *Managing Otitis Media with Effusion in Young Children*, provides a summary of diagnosis and hearing evaluation, environmental and risk factors, therapeutic interventions, and an algorithm for management. Table 1–4, from the AHCPR Guidelines, summarizes various outcomes in treatment of OME. The AHCPR Guidelines may be summarized as follows:

- Hearing evaluation is recommended when OME persists for more than three months.
- If bilateral hearing loss greater than 20 dB HL is present, treatment options include antibiotic therapy or tympanostomy tube placement, and control of environmental factors.

TABLE 1-4 Summary of potential benefits and risks of various interventions for treatment of OME. Assumes an otherwise healthy child with no craniofacial, neurologic, or sensory deficits.

Intervention	Potential Benefits	Potential Risks
Antibiotics	Improved clearance of effusion at one month or less. Possible reduction in future infections.	Nausea, vomiting, diarrhea (2%–32% depending on dose and antibiotic). Cutaneous reactions ($\leq$5%) Cost. Possible development of resistant strains of bacteria.
Antibiotics plus steroids	Possible improved clearance at one month (25.1%). Possible reduction in future infections.	See antibiotics and steroids separately.
Steroids alone	Possible improved clearance at one month (4.5%).	Possible exacerbation of varicella. Long-term complications not established for low doses. Cost.
Antihistamine/ decongestant	No apparent benefits.	Drowsiness and/or excitability. Cost.
Myringotomy with tubes	Immediate clearance of effusion in all children. Improved hearing.	Invasive procedure. Anesthesia risk. Cost. Otorrhea Possible restrictions on swimming.
Adenoidectomy	Benefits for young children have not been established.	Invasive procedure. Anesthesia risk. Cost.
Tonsillectomy	No apparent benefits.	Invasive procedure. Anesthesia risk. Cost.

Adapted from "Otitis media with effusion in young children. Clinical practice guideline, Number 12," by S. E. Stool et al., 1994, AHCPR Publication No. 94–0622. Rockville, MD: Agency for Health Care Policy and Research, Public Health Service, U.S. Department of Health and Human Services.

- Tympanostomy tubes and environmental modifications are recommended for any child with OME lasting 4–6 months accompanied by bilateral hearing loss (greater than 20 dB HL).

"Environmental modifications," in this context, refer to improvements in the acoustic environment that result in improved receptive communication for the child. These modifications may range from preferential seating to the use of an assistive listening device.

It is important to note that OME is more likely to escape detection than acute otitis media because the child with OME is usually asymptomatic except for the temporary hearing loss caused by the middle ear effusion. Thus, screening procedures are generally aimed at the identification of OME. Without systematic screening efforts, identification of OME is likely to be delayed or missed entirely.

Disorders of the Inner Ear

Most inner ear disease is permanent and irreversible. It may be present at birth or it may occur with sudden onset or gradual progression. Damage to the cochlea can occur from many causes, both pre- and postnatal (see Table 1–5).

Congenital causes may be genetic in origin, occurring alone or in association with other abnormalities (syndromes). When congenital deafness does not have a genetic origin it may occur alone, casued by premature birth and anoxia (oxygen deprivation), or it may be associated with other prenatal abnormalities such as *maternal rubella*. Inner ear disease and associated hearing loss can also be acquired after birth as a result of postnatal infection (e.g., meningitis, syphilis, or viral infection), ototoxic drugs, tumors, or trauma to the ear. Certain conditions place newborn infants and young children at increased risk for permanent hearing loss. The risk indicators compiled by the Joint Committee on Infant Hearing (2000) are summarized in Table 1–6 (see Appendix for complete text of JCIH 2000 Position Statement).

The prevalence of hearing loss from inner ear disease is low in comparison to hearing loss from middle ear disease, but high in comparison to other disorders routinely screened at birth. In fact, hearing loss is the most common birth disorder to occur in newborn infants. For example, hearing loss is 20 times more prevalent than phenylketonuria (PKU), a condition for which newborns have been screened for many years. The prevalence of permanent hearing loss in all newborn infants is approximately 3 per 1,000 births. For infants with one or more high risk factors, the prevalence of congenital hearing loss is at least ten times higher. This results in approximately 33 babies born each day (12,000 per year) in the United States with permanent hearing loss.

Disorders of the Auditory Nerve and Central Pathway

In children, *auditory neuropathy* or a *central auditory processing disorder* may exist. Auditory neuropathy and related neural conduction disorders refer to conditions where behavioral or physiologic measures suggest significant hearing loss, yet measures of cochlear function, specifically outer hair cell function, appear normal. Auditory neuropathy has only recently been described, and neither its etiology nor its natural history are well understood at this time.

TABLE 1-5 Causes of sensory hearing loss in children.

	Prenatal Causes
Genetic disorders	Nonsyndromic hereditary
	• May be autosomal recessive; autosomal dominant; X-linked
	Syndromic hereditary
	• Waardenburg syndrome (autosomal dominant)
	• Jervell and Lange-Nielsen syndrome
	• Usher syndrome (autosomal recessive)
	• Pendred syndrome (autosomal recessive)
	• Bronchio-oto-renal syndrome (autosomal dominant)
	• Stickler syndrome (autosomal dominant)
	• Alport Syndrome (autosomal dominant or X-linked; delayed onset HL)
	Chromosomal abnormalities (Trisomy 13; 18; 21)
	Inner ear malformations (e.g., Michel's, Mondini's, Scheibe's)
Intrauterine exposure	Infection
	• Syphilis
	• Toxoplasmosis
	• Cytomegalic inclusion disease (especially with primary viral infection, CMV)
	• Rubella
	• Herpes
	• Fetal alcohol syndrome
	Teratogens (external agents that can cause abnormal development)
	• Streptomycin
	• Quinine
	• Chloroquine phosphate
	• Thalidomides
	Postnatal Causes
Infection	Meningitis
	Labyrinthitis (measles, mumps, herpes zoster)
Trauma	Anoxia
	Premature birth
	Temporal bone fracture
	Noise
	• Explosive noise
	• Repeated exposure to loud noise (e.g., NICU incubators)
Ototoxic medications	Aminoglycosides (e.g., gentamicin, kanamycin, neomycin, tobramycin)
	Loop diuretics
	Chemotherapeutic agents (e.g., cisplatin)

Moreover, the term is probably too narrow to encompass the range of auditory neural and/or brainstem conduction disorders that produce these findings.

TABLE 1-6 Joint Committee on Infant Hearing Year 2000 Position Statement: High-risk indicators for hearing loss in neonates and infants.

A. Risk Criteria: Neonates (birth–28 days)

An illness or condition requiring admission to a neonatal intensive care unit for a period of 48 hours or more.

Stigmata or other findings associated with a syndrome known to include a sensorineural and/or conductive hearing loss.

Family history of permanent childhood sensorineural hearing loss.

Craniofacial anomalies, including those with morphological abnormalities of the pinna and ear canal.

In-utero infection such as cytomegalovirus, herpes, toxoplasmosis, or rubella.

B. Risk Criteria: Infants (29 days–2 years)

These indicators place an infant at risk for progressive or delayed-onset sensorineural hearing loss and/or conductive hearing loss:

Parental or caregiver concern regarding hearing, speech, language, and/or developmental delay.

Family history of permanent childhood hearing loss.

Stigmata or other findings associated with a syndrome known to include a sensorineural or conductive hearing loss or Eustachian tube dysfunction.

Postnatal infections associated with sensorineural hearing loss including bacterial meningitis.

In-utero infections such as cytomegalovirus, herpes, rubella, syphilis, and toxoplasmosis.

Neonatal indicators—specifically, hyperbilirubinemia at a serum level requiring exchange transfusion, persistent pulmonary hypertension of the newborn associated with mechanical ventilation, and conditions requiring the use of extracorporeal membrane oxygenation (ECMO).

Syndromes associated with progressive hearing loss, such as neurofibromatosis, osteopetrosis, and Usher syndrome.

Neurodegenerative disorders, such as Hunter syndrome, or sensory motor neuropathies such as Friedreich's ataxia and Charcot-Marie-Tooth syndrome.

Head trauma.

Recurrent or persistent otitis media with effusion for at least three months.

Research is ongoing to determine the prevalence of these disorders and how they should be approached with regard to identification and treatment. Most infant hearing screening programs are not designed to identify auditory neuropathy at birth, although this may change as more is learned about the disorder. It now appears that children with histories of hyperbilirubinemia and other illnesses requiring neonatal intensive care, are at increased risk for auditory neuropathy and other conditions that affect the central auditory nervous system. The risk of auditory neuropathy or brainstem pathway dysfunction also appears to be higher for infants with neurogenerative, neurometabolic, or demyelinating diseases. Thus, when screening these children some programs are electing to apply methods more likely to identify auditory neuropathy (see Chapter 2).

Central auditory processing disorders (CAPD) are functional disorders resulting from disease, trauma, or developmental abnormalities of the central auditory nervous system in children. CAPD is usually *idiopathic* and may be difficult to distinguish from disorders of receptive language processing, auditory memory, or attention. CAPD assessment usually consists of a battery of behavioral and physiologic tests, some of which require considerable motivation and concentration on the part of the test subject. For that reason, CAPD assessment is usually undertaken with children over the age of five years, who are suspected of having the disorder based on behavioral observation. Diagnosis and intervention planning for CAPD is best accomplished by a multidisciplinary team that includes an audiologist, speech-language pathologist, educational specialist, neuropsychologist, and developmental pediatrician.

THE NATURE OF HEARING LOSS

Peripheral hearing loss, caused by a disorder of the outer, middle, or inner ear, can be categorized as either *conductive* or *sensorineural*. Hearing loss that is both sensorineural and conductive in nature is referred to as a *mixed* hearing loss. As noted above, when an auditory disorder exists but the outer, middle, and inner ear mechanisms are functioning normally, the impairment is categorized as a central auditory processing disorder.

Conductive hearing loss occurs when there is a disease of the external ear canal, tympanic membrane, or middle ear, which interferes with the transmission of sound along the normal air conduction pathway. Conductive impairment is characterized by hearing loss for air-conducted sounds; however, the sounds conveyed directly to the inner ear via bone conduction are minimally affected. Conductive hearing loss can often be treated successfully, either with medication or surgical intervention.

Sensorineural hearing loss occurs when there is damage to the sensory cells of the cochlea or the fibers of the auditory nerve. In children, cochlear impairment is usually associated with one or more of the high-risk factors in Table 1–6 or caused by recessive genetic factors. Pure neural disorders, such as tumors on the auditory nerve, are far less common than sensory disorders, especially in children. Thus, most hearing losses described as sensorineural are, in fact, sensory (cochlear) in origin. Sensorineural hearing loss cannot be identified by physical examination because the external auditory canal and the tympanic membrane appear normal. Although most sensorineural losses are not amenable to medical treatment, almost everyone with sensorineural loss can benefit from hearing aid use. Those with hearing loss too severe to benefit from hearing aid use may be candidates for a *cochlear implant.*

Hearing loss is also described according to whether the loss is *unilateral* (one ear affected) or *bilateral* (both ears affected). The developmental consequences of bilateral hearing loss have been demonstrated in many studies, but it was once believed that unilateral hearing loss had no effect on language development and learning. While in many cases this appears to be true, there is now evidence that a substantial number of children with unilateral hearing loss are delayed in their language and academic performance. Consequently, children with unilateral hearing loss need regular monitoring so that parents and school personnel may be advised of the need for special services, preferential seating or, in some cases, fitting of an appropriate hearing aid or assistive listening device. Furthermore, preservation of hearing in the normal ear must be strongly encouraged.

The *degree* of hearing loss must also be determined. The degree of loss is generally expressed as an average in decibels Hearing Level (dB HL). This is commonly expressed as a *pure-tone average* based on the air conduction thresholds at 500 Hz, 1000 Hz, and 2000 Hz. Although descriptive terms commonly used to categorize degrees of hearing loss vary considerably, the following are typical:

- normal (0–15 dB HL)
- slight hearing loss (16–25 dB HL)
- mild hearing loss (26–45 dB HL)
- moderate hearing loss (46–75 dB HL)
- severe hearing loss (76–100 dB HL)
- profound hearing loss (100+dB HL).

IMPLICATIONS OF HEARING LOSS AND OTITIS MEDIA

The effects of bilateral sensorineural hearing loss in children are well documented. Even a *mild* bilateral sensorineural hearing loss can have significant consequences. Permanent hearing loss in young children almost always affects the development of speech and language, and often academic performance and social-emotional development as well. Although most deaf and hard-of-hearing adults are productive, well-adjusted members of society, hearing loss can have a detrimental effect on interpersonal relationships and career opportunities. Fortunately, early identification and intervention combined with the use of hearing aids and other sensory devices can significantly reduce the impact of sensorineural hearing loss on a young child. Early identification of hearing loss is crucial so that families can make well-informed decisions about intervention and audiologic management. Some will make choices aimed at maximizing the use of residual hearing, oral language, and speech production. Indeed, infants can now be fitted with amplification soon after the hearing loss is identified. Other families will choose sign language or a sign system for communication. Audiologists and professionals from related disciplines play a key role in providing the information families need to select an intervention plan well suited to their goals and preferences.

In general, the greater the degree of hearing loss, the greater the implications for oral language development. However, research has shown that children who are identified and given appropriate intervention before six months of age maintain language development consistent with their cognitive abilities, at least through the age of five years, regardless of their degree of hearing loss. Apart from the age of identification, degree of hearing loss, or age of intervention, it is important to remember that each child is an individual whose unique characteristics and environment will interact to determine the consequences of a hearing loss.

The implications of otitis media and conductive hearing loss are less clear than those associated with sensorineural hearing loss. Although rare, untreated chronic otitis media can result in serious medical complications that include *cholesteatoma, meningitis,* and sensorineural hearing loss. Far more common is persistent conductive hearing loss caused by the presence of middle ear effusion. While the implications are not fully understood, behavioral and electrophysiologic studies have shown that persistent conductive hearing loss secondary to OME early in life may be associated with reduced auditory processing ability, particularly at the level of the brainstem. Interestingly, some of these effects are observed even after hearing sensitivity has returned to normal. Similarly, some children with histories of persistent or recurrent OME show reduced understanding of speech in the presence of competing noise, even after auditory thresholds and middle ear function return to normal. The effects of OME on speech, language, and learning have been investigated for many years. Findings have been mixed, with some studies indicating a relationship between persistent OME and reduced language skills or school performance. Others have found no significant association or one that is related only indirectly. While specific cause and effect relationships remain under investigation, it is widely recognized that persistent or recurrent OME has potentially detrimental long-term consequences, especially for children already experiencing communicative disorders related to learning disabilities or developmental delays. Thus, it is important to systematically screen for OME so that children whose conditions require medical, audiologic, or speech-language intervention can be identified and appropriately treated.

PRINCIPLES OF SCREENING

The purpose of screening is to identify those individuals most likely to have a disorder or condition from among a group of people with no apparent symptoms. For each screening outcome there are costs as well as benefits. In general, costs are determined by: 1) the number of individuals who actually have the condition in proportion to the total number screened, 2) the expenses associated with the screening process, and 3) the number of incorrect screening outcomes. Benefits, on the other hand, are generally associated with *correct* screening outcomes.

A *true positive* occurs when the target condition is correctly identified. This outcome is obviously beneficial because treatment that otherwise might have been denied or delayed can be provided. Screening can also result in a *true negative*; that is, a negative screening outcome in an individual who is truly free of the condition. A true negative is beneficial because the family can be assured of the condition's absence. A *false positive* occurs when the screening results indicate the need for referral but subsequent diagnostic tests indicate the absence of the condition. This outcome can be expensive from a financial standpoint because it entails unnecessary follow-up. It is also costly in human terms if individuals or their families are needlessly concerned or inconvenienced. Finally, a *false negative* occurs when the screening procedure indicates a pass even though the disorder is, in fact, present. This is considered the most serious error because the screening procedure fails to uncover an existing disorder. The costs associated with a false negative may be financial (inappropriate intervention or educational placement) as well as emotional (families are given erroneous information).

To determine the performance of a screening protocol it is necessary to calculate its *validity*. Several terms developed in the field of clinical epidemiology are useful in this regard. The first is *prevalence*, which is defined as the number of cases of a disease existing in a given population during a specified time period (period prevalence) or at a particular point in time (point prevalence). A related term sometimes mistakenly used interchangeably is *incidence*. Incidence is defined as the number of new cases identified over a given period of time, usually one year. Recall that otitis media is a highly prevalent disease, affecting nearly all children at least once during the early months or years of life. The incidence may vary, however, depending on the time of year. In contrast, sensorineural hearing loss occurs far less frequently than otitis media, with an incidence of approximately 3 per 1,000 for all newborn infants and an incidence of over 30 per 1,000 for babies with one or more of the conditions listed in Table 1–6.

In addition to considering the incidence or prevalence of a disorder, determining the validity of a screening procedure requires determination of *sensitivity* and *specificity*. *Sensitivity* refers to the number of people with a given disorder who test positive; that is, the rate of correct classification for affected individuals. It is calculated by dividing the number of true positives by the sum of the true positives and false negatives, or:

$$\text{Sensitivity} = \frac{\text{True Positives}}{\text{True Positives} + \text{False Negatives}} \times 100\%$$

Thus, if 100 infants have a hearing loss and the test is able to identify 90 of them, the test has a sensitivity of 90%.

In contrast, *specificity* refers to the test's accuracy in correctly identifying persons who *do not* have the condition; that is, the rate of correct classification for unaffected individuals. It is calculated by dividing the number of true negatives by the sum of the true negatives and false positives, or:

$$\text{Specificity} = \frac{\text{True Negatives}}{\text{True Negatives} + \text{False Positives}} \times 100\%$$

Thus, if 100 babies have normal hearing and the screening test is able to classify 90 of them as normal, the test has a specificity of 90%.

It should be obvious that the ideal screening test would have both high sensitivity and high specificity, meaning that false-negatives (misses) as well as false-positives (unnecessary referrals) would be few. There is an important trade-off, however, between sensitivity and specificity, the extent of which is determined by the pass-fail criteria, that is, the rules that define a pass or a fail on a given screening test. The relationship between sensitivity and specificity is illustrated in Figure 1–9. This figure shows two hypothetical distributions, one representing individuals without the disorder of interest (A) and the other representing those with the disorder (B). In this example, the two groups have very different screening outcomes. As is typical of most screening scenarios, there are many people without the disorder in comparison to those who have it. Also, affected individuals show greater variability in their test results. In the figure, population A, with no disorder, exhibits hypothetical screening results ranging from approximately 2 to 16. Population B, the group with the disorder, exhibits hypothetical screening results ranging from approximately 10 to 30. Note that the two distributions overlap from 10 to 16, meaning that there are a few individuals without the disorder whose screening outcome measures were unusually

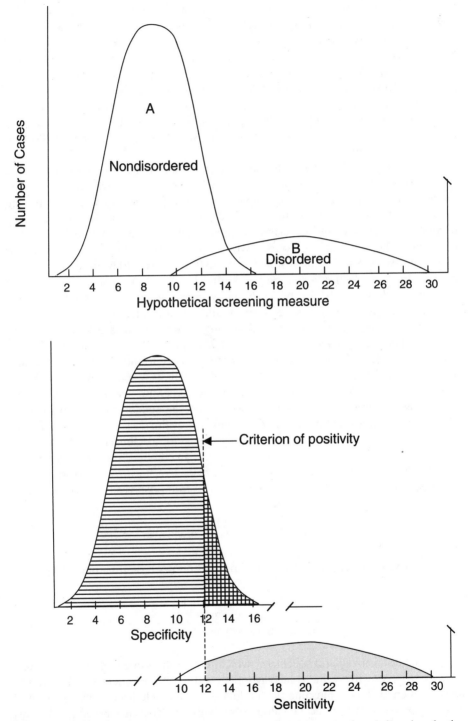

Figure 1-9 Two distributions showing overlapping normal and disordered subjects and illustrating the relationship between sensitivity and specificity. (Adapted from *Principles and procedures in the evaluation of screening for disease*, by R. Thorner and Q. Remein, 1971, National Center for Health Services Research and Development.)

high, and a few with the disorder whose measures were unusually low. If the criterion for a positive outcome were set at 12 as shown, people who have this value or higher when tested would be classified as positive, and thus referred for diagnostic follow-up. Note that using 12 as the criterion for referral would mean that disordered subjects with a test result lower than 12 would be missed (false negatives). The average sensitivity is represented by the shaded area in distribution B (true positives) divided by the total area of distribution B (true positives plus false negatives). The specificity would be the striped area (true negatives) divided by the cross-hatched area, which is the total area of distribution A (true negatives plus false positives).

From Figure 1–9 it should be clear that sensitivity and specificity of a screening test will be altered according to where the examiner chooses to draw the line for pass and refer. For example, if the cutoff for a pass were 16 (moving the vertical bar to the right), the test would have 100% specificity since all truly normal individuals would be classified as normal (i.e., there would be no false positives). The trade-off, of course, would be low sensitivity, since disordered individuals whose screening results fall from 10 to 16 would also be classified as normal. In contrast, the screening test would have 100 percent sensitivity if the cutoff were drawn at 10. In this case, many more individuals without the disorder (false positives) would be referred for additional testing.

In assessing the validity of a screening procedure, it is also important to consider the *predictive value. Positive predictive value* (PPV) refers to the percentage of cases with positive screening outcomes that are found, by diagnostic evaluation, to actually have the disorder. Stated differently, PPV indicates the likelihood of the target condition being present when the screening test is positive. In contrast, *negative predictive value* refers to the percentage of cases with negative screening outcomes that are found, by diagnostic evaluation, to be free of the disorder. A test's predictive value is especially important to clinicians as their goal is to use the screening test to determine whether a given child has the disorder (*positive predictive value*) or does not have the disorder (*negative predictive value*). The PPV is calculated by dividing the number of true positives by all positives, or:

$$PPV = \frac{\text{True Positives}}{\text{True Positives} + \text{False Positives}} \times 100\%$$

The NPV is determined by dividing the number of true negatives by all negatives, or:

$$NPV = \frac{\text{True Negatives}}{\text{True Negatives} + \text{False Negatives}} \times 100\%$$

Unlike sensitivity and specificity, which remain the same regardless of disease prevalence, predictive value is heavily influenced by the prevalence of the disorder being screened. This is illustrated in Table 1–7, which includes calculation of sensitivity, specificity, and predictive value. Note that prevalence has no effect on sensitivity or specificity, while predictive value is greatly affected by prevalence.

Disorders with low prevalence are likely to have lower positive predictive value and higher negative predictive value. Thus, the rarer the disease, the lower the positive predictive value because the proportion of true positives is smaller.

TABLE 1-7 Performance of a hypothetical screening procedure (TEST) for identification of a hypothetical condition (DISEASE) in two groups differing only in prevalence (1% vs. 10%). The TEST has a sensitivity (SENS) of 90% and specificity (SPEC) of 85% in both groups; however, note the effect of disease prevalence on the positive predictive value (PPV) and the negative predictive value (NPV) in the two groups and the number of false positives that occur.

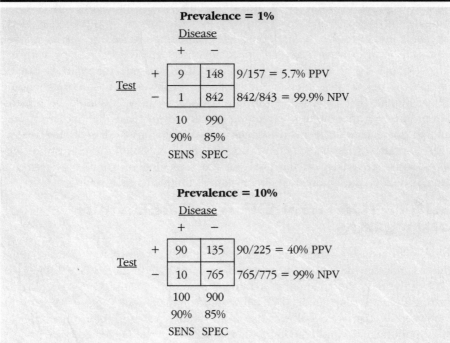

Prevalence = 1%

Disease

		+	−	
Test	+	9	148	9/157 = 5.7% PPV
	−	1	842	842/843 = 99.9% NPV
		10	990	
		90%	85%	
		SENS	SPEC	

Prevalence = 10%

Disease

		+	−	
Test	+	90	135	90/225 = 40% PPV
	−	10	765	765/775 = 99% NPV
		100	900	
		90%	85%	
		SENS	SPEC	

From "Critical issues in acoustic-immittance screening for middle-ear effusion," by R.J. Nozza, 1995, Seminars in Hearing, 16 (1), 86–98.

Similarly, the rarer the disease, the higher the negative predictive value because of the larger proportion of true negatives. Since the true status of each individual is unknown at the time of screening, knowledge of the predictive value for each screening procedure is critically important. Referring again to Figure 1–9, the positive predictive value is represented by the shaded area (true positives) divided by the sum of the shaded area plus the cross-hatched portion of distribution A (true positives plus false positives). Despite its importance, predictive value is perhaps the least understood screening principle. But without it, a screening protocol cannot be properly evaluated. Moreover, consideration only of sensitivity and specificity without regard to predictive value can result in a distorted view of how well a screening protocol is performing. To meaningfully apply measures of predictive value it is important to understand their relationship to sensitivity and specificity and what can be done to improve them. In particular, it is important to remember that the vast majority of individuals screened in any program will not have the target condition. Thus, the false positives are derived from this relatively large pool of individuals. Consequently, problems with low predictive value are usually caused by low specificity. Even a small reduction in specificity can result in a large decline in predictive value because the proportion of individuals without the disorder is so great. Thus, the goal is to increase sensitivity with minimal effect on specificity. There are at least two ways this might be accomplished. One way is to limit screening to those individuals already known to be at increased risk. The disadvantage, in the context of infant hearing screening, is that no more than half of the infants with congenital hearing loss have high risk factors. Thus, improving positive predictive value would occur at the expense of lower sensitivity. A more favorable approach is to do repeated measures or a multiple-stage screening procedure. A two-stage approach, used in many screening programs, may involve rescreening with the same technology or a different technology. If the number of referrals can be lowered by rescreening, then the rate of false positives and the corresponding specificity and predictive value will improve significantly. It should be remembered, however, that multiple screening procedures increase the amount of time and, in some cases, the instrumentation required, thus adding to the overall costs associated with the screening program. Each of these factors must be carefully considered based on the goals of the screening program, the costs and benefits derived, and individual circumstances unique to each setting.

JUSTIFICATION OF A SCREENING PROGRAM

In order to justify the time and resources required for a comprehensive screening program, several important prerequisites must be considered (see Table 1–8). Most of the requisite conditions in Table 1–8 are easily satisfied in screening for hearing loss and otitis media, but a few issues remain controversial. Most of the controversies, discussed below, arise from differences of opinion regarding the costs, both financial and emotional, in comparison to the perceived benefits.

Universal Newborn Hearing Screening

Approximately four million babies are born each year in the United States and about 10% have one or more conditions that increase their risk for hearing loss. Studies have revealed that screening only those infants identified as high risk will identify only about half of all babies born with permanent hearing loss. Obviously, early identification and intervention are important for all infants, not

---

TABLE 1-8 General prerequisites for a screening program.

1. The problem is significant to the individual and to society.
2. There is good evidence of effective treatment once the problem is detected.
3. The screening test has been properly evaluated and shown to be acceptable in the setting where screening is to be performed.
4. There is evidence that a screening program resulting in treatment is of greater benefit than waiting until symptoms develop.
5. Cost issues have been considered and judged to be reasonable.
6. There are plausible strategies and sufficient resources to ensure implementation.

Adapted with permission from "Screening in the 1990's: Some principles and guidelines," by J.W. Feightner, 1999, in Screening Children for Auditory Function *(Chapter 1, pp. 1–16), by F.H. Bass and J.W. Hall (eds.), 1999, Nashville, TN: Bill Wilkerson Center Press.*

just those with high risk factors. Identification of the other 50% of infants with congenital hearing loss necessitates "universal hearing screening," the screening of all newborn infants. This is an ambitious goal, but one that has been promoted by several governmental and professional organizations, including the National Institute on Deafness and Other Communication Disorders (1993), a branch of the National Institutes of Health, and the Joint Committee on Infant Hearing (JCIH), a multidisciplinary organization that includes audiologists, physicians, educators of the deaf, early intervention specialists, and consumers (see Appendix). Screening for hearing loss in the first month is also advocated by the U.S. Public Health Service's "Healthy People 2000" initiative and its 2010 health objectives. Contained within these initiatives are recommendations that infants be seen for diagnostic follow-up by three months, and enrolled in appropriate intervention services by six months of age. In order to reflect the continuum of interdisciplinary services needed to deliver a comprehensive program of infant hearing screening, many organizations now refer to the process of hearing screening and follow up as Early Hearing Detection and Intervention (EHDI). The Joint Committee on Infant Hearing Year 2000 Position Statement sets forth eight principles intended to serve as a foundation for EHDI programs.[1]

1. All infants have access to hearing screening using a physiologic measure. Newborns who receive routine care have access to hearing screening during their hospital birth admission. Newborns in alternative birthing facilities, including home births, have access to and are referred for screening before one month of age. All newborns or infants who require neonatal intensive care receive hearing screening before discharge from the hospital. These components constitute universal newborn hearing screening (UNHS).
2. All infants who do not pass the birth admission screen and any subsequent rescreening begin appropriate audiologic and medical evaluations to confirm the presence of hearing loss before three months of age.
3. All infants with confirmed permanent hearing loss receive services before six months of age in interdisciplinary intervention programs that recognize and build on strengths, informed choice, traditions, and cultural beliefs of the family.
4. All infants who pass newborn hearing screening but who have risk indicators for other auditory disorders and/or speech and language delay receive ongoing audiologic and medical surveillance and monitoring for communication development. Infants with indicators associated with late-onset, progressive, or fluctuating hearing loss as well as auditory neural conduction disorders and/or brainstem auditory pathway dysfunction should be monitored.
5. Infant and family rights are guaranteed through informed choice, decision-making, and consent.
6. Infant hearing screening and evaluation results are afforded the same protection as all other health care and educational information. As new standards for privacy and confidentiality are proposed, they must balance the needs of society and the rights of the infant and family, without compromising the ability of health and education to provide care.

---

[1]These principles are accompanied by specific benchmarks and quality indicators. See Appendix for full text of the JCIH Year 2000 Position Statement.

7. Information systems are used to measure and report the effectiveness of EHDI services. While state registries measure and track screening, evaluation, and intervention outcomes for infants and their families, efforts should be made to honor a family's privacy by removing identifying information wherever possible. Aggregate state and national data may also be used to measure and track the impact of EHDI programs on public health and education while maintaining the confidentiality of individual infant and family information.
8. EHDI programs provide data to monitor quality, demonstrate compliance with legislation and regulations, determine fiscal accountability and cost effectiveness, support reimbursement for services, and mobilize and maintain community support (JCIH Year 2000 Position Statement, page 9).

Fortunately, permanent hearing loss occurs rarely in young children, but its relatively low incidence makes it challenging to design cost-effective screening models. Recall that conditions with low prevalence are often associated with screening outcomes that have low predictive value even though sensitivity and specificity may be high. Current methods of infant hearing screening have excellent sensitivity (close to 100%); thus, a child with a permanent hearing loss is rarely missed. But the same screening methods are somewhat less accurate with respect to correctly identifying normal hearing individuals at the time of screening. Consequently, many babies referred for follow-up turn out to have normal hearing. Consider, for example, a state with 100,000 births per year and a hearing-screening program with an impressive pass rate of 98%. If 100,000 were screened, 98,000 babies would pass and 2,000 would be referred for follow up. But among the 2000 referred, even if we assume a relatively high incidence of 5:1,000 for all degrees of hearing loss, only 10 would turn out to have permanent hearing loss while 1,990 would have normal hearing (or transient conductive hearing loss secondary to middle ear effusion). This example highlights two challenges of infant hearing screening: 1) the low incidence of permanent hearing loss means that the number of children identified will be small in proportion to the number screened; and 2) the relatively low positive predictive value means that only a fraction of the children referred will turn out to have permanent hearing loss. The first issue, low incidence, is important because it implies that universal screening programs are relatively expensive if considered in terms of cost per child identified. The second issue, low positive predictive value, is important because it means that some families will be unnecessarily concerned or inconvenienced. Consequently, policy makers are justified in asking whether universal hearing screening is, in fact, worth the time and expense. In response, advocates have argued convincingly in support of universal hearing screening (see Table 1–9). Indeed, there is compelling evidence of improved developmental outcomes for children and their families when hearing loss is detected soon after birth and intervention is begun at an early age. Furthermore, if early identification and intervention reduce the need for special education and rehabilitation services, infant hearing screening can be argued in fiscal terms as well.

EHDI programs are expanding rapidly throughout the nation. Most states have passed legislation to mandate newborn hearing screening, and federal legislation is providing financial resources to support these efforts in many states. Still, ongoing evaluation is needed to better understand the advantages of early

TABLE 1-9 Justification for newborn infant hearing screening.
1. Hearing loss is sufficiently prevalent to warrant screening; indeed, it is considerably more prevalent than several other diseases routinely screened at birth;
2. The sequelae of hearing loss are sufficient to merit newborn screening, as evidenced by the developmental delays imposed by hearing loss as well as the relatively higher cost of late identification;
3. Accurate, efficient, and cost effective screening procedures are available;
4. Early detection appears to result in better long-term developmental outcomes;
5. Intervention services are available and even mandated by law; and
6. The cost of infant hearing screening is commensurate with the benefits derived.

From Northern, J. and Hayes, D., 1996

identification as well as the best methods of achieving accurate detection of hearing loss, while minimizing the impact on families whose children have normal hearing.

Screening for Hearing Loss in High-Risk Infants

As noted earlier, about 10% of all newborn infants have one or more high-risk conditions and studies have shown that the incidence of permanent hearing loss in the high risk population ranges from 3–5%. Thus, for every 1000 high-risk babies screened, as many as 50 could be found to have permanent hearing loss in one or both ears. Screening of high-risk infants for permanent hearing loss has been widely supported for many years because the relatively high incidence of permanent hearing loss in this population results in higher positive predictive value, making the cost per child identified considerably lower. In addition, the logistics of screening are simplified because many high-risk infants have health-related conditions that require a longer hospital stay. But as noted earlier, high-risk screening alone misses at least half of all infants with hearing loss. Furthermore, screening only in the high-risk nursery poses additional challenges to follow-up, as infants are usually transferred to their local hospitals, often far from the tertiary facility where hearing screening was performed. For these reasons, the JCIH Year 2000 Position Statement no longer recommends screening at-risk infants, but instead advocates the screening of *all* newborn infants. The risk factors compiled in Table 1–6 are useful where universal hearing screening programs are not yet established, or for the purpose of identifying infants needing continued surveillance because of risks associated with delayed onset or acquired hearing loss.

Screening for Hearing Loss in Older Children

Mass screening for hearing loss in preschool and school-age children has been practiced for many years. It has not been controversial because the costs associated with this activity are relatively low. Furthermore, since many young children are enrolled in group preschool programs and nearly all are eventually enrolled in public or private schools, the screening protocols and logistics of identification, rescreening, and follow-up are time consuming but relatively uncomplicated. Unfortunately, school-age hearing screening programs are sometimes poorly organized and conducted by unqualified screening personnel.

Screening for Otitis Media

Screening for otitis media has been controversial but for different reasons than those associated with hearing screening. Although the prevalence of otitis media among infants and toddlers is high compared to the prevalence of permanent hearing loss in children, middle ear problems are highly transient. Thus, a child who tests positive on the screening day may have no apparent problem when seen later for medical examination. Furthermore, it is not clear whether mild hearing loss secondary to OME is harmful to young children. Studies showing both positive and negative associations have been reported in the literature. It is important to note, however, that most of the longitudinal studies have examined children whose development is typical in most respects. Hearing loss in a child who is already experiencing developmental delays is likely to create an added burden. Even so, the benefits of middle ear screening are frequently questioned. As with hearing screening, the efficacy of middle ear screening must be judged by considering the relative costs and benefits. In this context it is important to recognize that otitis media, even in the form of OME, is an abnormal condition that warrants medical review even though the physician may choose not to treat it. Serious medical complications from otitis media are rare but examination by a physician is needed to determine the appropriate course of action. It should also be emphasized that OME accompanied by hearing loss has potential implications beyond the realm of medical management since children who respond abnormally to speech and other sounds are often described as inattentive, asocial, or developmentally delayed. Because of these concerns, screening for OME should include a combined protocol consisting of hearing and middle ear screening.

CONFIDENTIALITY, INFORMED CONSENT, AND LIABILITY

It was noted earlier that parental permission must be obtained prior to conducting hearing and middle ear screening procedures, unless consent has already been obtained as part of an institutional enrollment process. Failure to ensure informed consent is not only unprofessional, but personnel and their institutions risk negative public relations and possible legal action. Parents have a right to be informed of all screening procedures and their purpose. They must also be protected from public discussion or distribution of screening outcomes without their knowledge and consent. Every screening program must have, as part of its procedural guidelines, a strict code of ethics regarding patient confidentiality. In many settings where hearing and middle ear screening are performed, institutional and/or accreditation guidelines will already exist. Screening personnel must be familiar with these policies and maintain full compliance at all times.

In addition to protecting the legal rights of patients and families, clinicians themselves must avoid liability. The risk of harm associated with routine hearing and middle ear screening is low. Even so, personnel must have liability insurance, either through their own policies or, more commonly, through their employers. In addition to personal liability, clinicians and their employers must protect themselves from liability associated with a missed identification. This is most likely to occur when a newborn infant does not get screened prior to discharge. The best legal protection in such cases is to provide clear communication with families regarding recommendations for follow-up and careful documentation of each contact. A software tracking and documentation procedure described in Chapter 6 provides a useful example of how this can be accomplished, even in a large-scale screening program.

PROGRAM EVALUATION

Programs must engage in critical, on-going self-examination of their screening outcomes. Failure to identify OME or hearing loss may result in lack of treatment or inappropriate decisions regarding educational placement or classification. But over-identification can lead to wasted resources as well as dissatisfied parents and health care providers. Although there is no universal standard for what constitutes a successful screening program, the JCIH Year 2000 Position Statement sets forth specific benchmarks and quality indicators for infant hearing screening. They include: 1) the percentage of infants screened during the birth admission, 2) the percentage of infants screened before one month of age, 3) the percentage of infants who do not pass the birth admission screen, 4) the percentage of infants who do not pass the birth admission screening who return for follow-up services, 5) the percentage of infants who do not pass the birth admission/outpatient screen/s who are referred for audiologic and medical evaluation, and 6) the percentage of families who refuse hearing screening on birth admission.

Final decisions regarding pass-fail criteria should be made by the supervising audiologist in consultation with other members of the screening team, as well as with service providers to whom referrals will be made. This requires the time and effort necessary to determine referral outcomes and their dispositions. While most programs do not have the necessary resources to engage in formal research, it is important for individual programs to track screening outcomes. An example is provided in Table 1–10 from Pitt County Community Hospital, a hospital in eastern North Carolina that uses automated auditory brainstem response testing to screen all newborn infants. Data are presented here for benchmark #3, above. Note that referral rates improved dramatically from 1996 to 1999 as improvements were made in technique and methodology. The data now show

TABLE 1-10 Screening outcomes for infants screened during birth admission, using automated ABR in a well-baby nursery, at a hospital in eastern North Carolina (personal communication, Rhonda Joyner, Pitt County Memorial Hospital, April 2000).

	1996	1997	1998	1999
Number of Infants Screened	2,438	2,486	2,833	2,783
% of Infants Passed	89.0	96.0	98.2	99.4
% of Infants Referred	11.0	4.0	1.8	<1

an impressive pass rate that exceeds 99%. Maximizing the initial pass rate is crucial since many of the children referred for follow-up will turn out to have normal hearing.

SUMMARY

Hearing disorders may occur at any age at all levels of the auditory system. Dysfunction at the level of the outer or middle ear results in a conductive hearing loss. Some conductive disorders, like otitis media, are highly prevalent in children. Others, such as those associated with congenital anomalies of the external ear or ossicles, are rare. Most conductive impairments can be successfully treated by a pediatrician or otolaryngologist, but chronic or undetected middle ear problems can have serious consequences. Thus, screening for OME in young children is essential.

When the disorder is at the level of the inner ear, the resulting sensory hearing loss is usually caused by cochlear dysfunction. Nearly all cochlear impairments are permanent and irreversible. Any degree of sensory hearing loss in children, whether unilateral or bilateral, needs to be identified and appropriately managed. Detection and intervention for sensory hearing loss in children is essential to prevent or minimize developmental delays.

Although rare, disorders of neural conduction or auditory brainstem pathway dysfunction can occur. In some cases these conditions are present at birth, although their natural history is not well understood at this time. Most programs do not attempt to screen for these disorders, but they may be uncovered in the process of hearing screening or diagnostic follow-up. As more is learned about auditory neuropathy and other neural conduction disorders, future screening may target these conditions as well.

Several assumptions and prerequisites to screening were discussed in this chapter. Among the most import is the establishment of validity. The validity of a screening procedure is determined by calculating the sensitivity, specificity, and predictive value of a given procedure, alone or in combination with other tests. In general, increasing the sensitivity occurs at the expense of lower specificity. In addition, it is important to consider predictive value, which indicates the likelihood of the target condition being present or absent when the screening test is positive or negative. Most screening programs do not have the resources to conduct formal investigations of validity but all are encouraged (and in some states are required) to collect their own data according to established guidelines and quality indicators.

Undetected hearing loss or middle ear disease in a child is always a serious matter. The need for early detection and follow-up is widely recognized. Even so, screening for hearing loss and otitis media have, at times, been controversial because of differences of opinion among professionals and health policy administrators regarding the extent to which various prerequisites have been satisfied. Although there is growing evidence of improved developmental outcomes when hearing loss is identified early and managed effectively, the need for further investigation continues.

In the final analysis, the success of a screening program will be measured by many factors, including the screening methods employed, the qualifications of screening personnel, and the effectiveness of communication with families and other professionals. For most screening programs, a formal research protocol that includes a "gold standard" for hearing loss or middle ear effusion is not feasible. Consequently, professionals engaged in hearing and middle ear screening must stay current with the professional literature so that findings of large-scale population studies and their implications can be considered in the design and implementation of a screening program. Part II of this text provides a description of how several programs successfully screen children at various ages in a variety of settings, using currently available instrumentation and methodology. Part III examines special considerations pertaining to referral, follow-up, and communication with families.

REFERENCES

Agency for Health Care Policy and Research. (1995). *Using clinical practice guidelines to evaluate quality of care* (Vol. 2, Methods, AHCPR Pub. No. 95–0046). Washington, DC: U.S. Department of Health and Human Services Public Health Service.

American Academy of Audiology (1997). Report and Position Statement: Identification of hearing loss and middle ear dysfunction in preschool and school-age children. *Audiology Today, 9,* (3) 18–23.

American Academy of Pediatrics (1999). Newborn and infant hearing loss: Detection and intervention. Task Force on Newborn and Infant Hearing. *Pediatrics, 103,* 527–530.

American Speech-Language-Hearing Association. (1997). *Guidelines for audiologic screening.* Rockville, MD: ASHA.

Arehart, K. H., Yoshinaga-Itano, C., Thomson, V., Gabbard, S. A., & Stredler-Brown, A. (1998). State of the states: The status of universal newborn screening, assessment, and intervention systems in 16 States. *American Journal of Audiology, 7,* 101–114.

Bess, F. H., & Tharpe, A. M. (1984). Unilateral hearing impairment in children. *Pediatrics, 74,* 206–216.

Bhatnagar, S. C. & Andy, O. J. (1995). *Neuroscience for the study of communicative disorders.* Baltimore: Williams & Wilkins.

Blair, J. C., Peterson, M. E., & Vieweg, S. H. (1985). The effects of mild sensorineural hearing loss on academic performance of young school-age children. *The Volta Review, 87* (2), 87–93.

Bluestone, C. D. & Klein, J. O. (1995). *Otitis media in infants and children.* Philadelphia: W.B. Saunders Company.

Bluestone, C. D., Klein, J. O., & Kenna, M. A., (Eds). *Pediatric otolaryngology* (Third ed.) Philadelphia: Saunders.

Daly, K. (1991). Epidemiology of otitis media. *Otolaryngol Clin N Am, 24,* 775–786.

Eddy, D. (1991). Common Screening Tests, Philadelphia: American College of Physicians

Feightner, J. W. (1992). Screening in the 1990's: Some principles and guidelines. In F. H. Bess and J. W. Hall (eds.) *Screening children for auditory function* (Chapter 1, pp. 1–16), Nashville: Bill Wilkerson Center Press.

Finitzo, T., Albright, K., & O'Neal, J. (1998). The newborn with hearing loss: Detection in the nursery. *Pediatrics, 102,* 1452–1460.

Friel-Patti, S., & Finitzo, T. (1990). Language learning in a prospective study of otitis media with effusion. *Journal of Speech Hearing Research, 33,* 188–194.

Gravel, J., Berg, A., Bradley, M., Cacace, A., Campbell, D., Dalzell, L., DeCristofaro, J., Greenberg, E., Gross, S., Orlando, M., Pinheiro, J., Regan, J., Spivak, L., Stevens, F., & Prieve, B. (2000). The New York State universal newborn hearing screening demonstration project: Effects of screening protocol on inpatient outcome measures. *Ear and Hearing, 21,* 131–140.

Harrison, M., & Roush, J. (1996). Age of suspicion, identification, and intervention for infants and young children with hearing loss: A national study. *Ear and Hearing 17,* 55–62.

Individuals with Disabilities Education Act Amendments of 1997, P.L. No. 105–17,111, Stat. 38 (1997). Codified as amended at 20 U.S.C. Section 1400–1485.

Joint Committee on Infant Hearing. (2000). Joint Committee on Infant Hearing: Year 2000 Position Statement. *Audiology Today,* August, Special Issue; 6-27.

Lucente, F. & Sobol, S. (1988). *Essentials of Otolaryngology.* New York: Raven Press.

Mehl, A. L., & Thomson, V. (1998). Newborn hearing screening: The great omission. *Pediatrics, 101,*

Meyerhoff, W. L. & Rice, D. H. (1992). *Otolaryngology—Head and neck surgery.* Philadelphia: W.B. Saunders Co.

National Institute on Deafness and Other Communication Disorders. (1993). National Institutes of Health Consensus Statement: *Early identification of hearing impairment in infants and young children.* Bethesda, MD: NIDOCD.

Northern, J. L. & Hayes, D. 1996. Universal screening for infant hearing impairment: Necessary, beneficial, and justifiable. *Audiology Today, 6* (3), 10–13.

Nozza, R. J. (1995). Critical issues in acoustic-immittance screening for middle-ear effusion. *Seminars in Hearing, 16* (1), 86–98.

Prieve, B., & Stevens, F. (2000). The New York State universal newborn hearing screening demonstration project: Introduction and overview. *Ear and Hearing, 21*, 85–91.

Rance, G., Beer, D. E., Cone-Wesson, B., Shepard, R. K., Dowell, R. C., King, A. M., Rickards, F. W., & Clark, G. M. (1999). Clinical findings for a group of infants and young children with auditory neuropathy. *Ear and Hearing, 20* (3), 238–252.

Roberts, J. E., Burchinal, M. R., Medley, L. P. (1995). Otitis media, hearing sensitivity, and maternal responsiveness in relation to language during infancy. *Journal of Pediatrics, 126*, 481–489.

Roush, J., & Matkin, N. D. (Eds.). (1994). *Infants and toddlers with hearing loss: Family-centered assessment and intervention.* Baltimore: York Press.

Ryan, A., & Dallos, P. (1984). Physiology of the Cochlea. In Northern, J. L. (ed): *Hearing Disorders* (Second ed.) (pp. 253–266). Boston: Little, Brown & Co.

Starr, A., Picton, T. W., Sininger, Y., Hood, L. J., & Berlin, C. I. (1996). Auditory neuropathy. *Brain, 119*, 741–753.

Stool, S. E., Berg, A. O., Berman, S., Carney, C. J., Cooley, J. R., Culpepper, L., Eavey R. D., Feagans, L. V., Finitzo, T., Friedman, E. (1994). *Managing otitis media with effusion in young children. Quick reference guide for clinicians* (AHCPR Publication 94–0623). Rockville, MD: Agency for Health Care Policy and Research, Public Health Service, U.S. Department of Health and Human Services.

Tharpe, A. M., & Clayton, E. W. (1997). Newborn hearing screening: Issues in legal liability and quality assurance. *American Journal of Audiology, 6*, 5–12.

Thorner, R. & Remein, Q. (1971). *Principles and procedures in the evaluation of screening for disease.* National Center for Health Services Research and Development, Dept. of Health, Education, and Welfare. Washington, DC: U.S. Government Printing Office.

U.S. Department of Education—Office of Special Education and Rehabilitative Services. (1998). *Final regulations: Early intervention program for infants and toddlers with disabilities.* Federal Register (34 CFR Part 303).

U.S. Department of Health and Human Services. (2000) Healthy People 2010 (Conference Edition, in Two Volumes). Washington, DC: U.S. Government Priority Office.

U.S. Department of Health and Human Services Public Health Service. (1990). *Healthy People 2000, National health promotion and disease prevention objectives for the nation* (DHHS Publication No. (PHS) 91–50212). Washington, DC: U.S. Government Printing Office.

Yoshinaga-Itano, C., Sedey, A., Coulter, D.K., & Mehl, A. L. (1998). Language of early and later identified children with hearing loss. *Pediatrics, 102*, 1161–1171.

Methods of Screening for Hearing Loss and Otitis Media

Jackson Roush

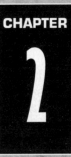

CHAPTER

2

INTRODUCTION

The purpose of screening is to identify children most likely to have a hearing or middle ear disorder in need of medical, audiologic, or speech-language intervention. It is important to clearly differentiate screening from diagnostic procedures. As noted in Chapter 1, screening is applied to populations with no apparent signs or symptoms of the target disorder. Diagnostic procedures are more expensive and time consuming than screening procedures and are, therefore, applied only when there is evidence of the disorder. Thus, the goal of a screening program is to identify asymptomatic individuals with an increased likelihood of having the target disorder, so that diagnostic procedures are applied only to that subset of individuals.

Most of the screening methods described in this chapter evolved from techniques originally developed for diagnostic purposes. As a result, screening usually involves an abbreviated or automated version of a more extensive procedure likely to be applied when individuals are referred for diagnostic evaluation. This chapter will focus primarily on screening methods; however, relevant diagnostic and specialized procedures will be highlighted in order to present the spectrum of test procedures used with children. Specifically, threshold measures, obtained with or without visual reinforcement audiometry should be provided only by an audiologist or under the direct supervision of an audiologist. It is important for non-audiologists to be aware of their "scope of practice" to ensure compliance with professional guidelines as well as state licensure laws and regulations. The procedures and protocols described in this chapter are consistent with guidelines and position statements of the American Academy of Audiology (1997) and the American Speech-Language-Hearing Association (1997).

PRELIMINARY CONSIDERATIONS

Many factors, most importantly the child's age and developmental status, influence the selection of a screening method. It is also necessary to determine whether the hearing-screening program will include screening for otitis media. In general, hearing status in neonates and young infants must be inferred from physiologic measures. Because physiologic procedures permit evaluation of the auditory system without the child's active participation, these procedures are often described as *objective hearing tests*. Once an infant reaches a developmental level of 5–6 months it is often possible to employ *behavioral hearing tests*, that is, those that involve observable responses. Detection of otitis media cannot be reliably accomplished using behavioral procedures but instead requires the use of physiologic procedures. Although various methods have been proposed for identification of otitis media, acoustic immittance measures are advocated in this text as the method of choice for detection of OME. Readers are encouraged to stay current with the literature regarding new methods of screening for otitis media. For example, *wide band acoustic reflectance* may prove to be useful for clinical assessment of middle ear status, especially in young infants. Also, otoacoustic emissions, described later in this chapter, hold considerable promise as a first-level screening procedure for both otitis media *and* hearing loss.

Institutional programs designed to screen children for hearing loss and otitis media generally occur in one of the following contexts: 1) mass (universal) hearing screening of newborns including well babies and those with high-risk factors; 2) hearing screening of "high-risk" infants in the neonatal intensive care unit or intermediate care nursery; 3) preschool hearing screening, which may or may not include screening for otitis media; and 4) school-based hearing screening, which typically includes screening for otitis media only at the lower elementary levels and for special populations. A fifth group, infants and toddlers from approximately 6 months to 3 years of age, have not historically been targeted for large-scale hearing screening because of the need for specialized personnel and instrumentation. Children in this age group are most often seen by an audiologist when parents or caretakers have concerns about hearing or when the child is being evaluated for concerns related to speech, language, or other developmental delays. As noted later in this chapter, however, the advent of otoacoustic emission screening has expanded the methodological options for detection of hearing loss in the infant/toddler population.

As noted in Chapter 1, screening of high-risk infants is uncontroversial because the higher incidence of permanent hearing loss in this population makes the cost per child identified easily justified. Only about 10% of all newborn infants have one or more high-risk conditions and the incidence of hearing loss is relatively high, between 3–5%. Physiologic screening of high-risk infants has been successfully practiced for many years. In contrast to high-risk screening, the appropriateness of universal infant hearing screening was controversial for many years, and to some degree still is. Recall from Chapter 1 that only about half of all infants born with permanent hearing loss have identifiable high-risk conditions. This means that a state with 100,000 births per year could identify about half of all newborns with congenital hearing loss just by screening the 10% (10,000) with high-risk indicators. But to identify all infants with congenital hearing loss it would be necessary to screen the other 90,000. This is an ambitious undertaking to be sure, but universal hearing screening programs are now in place throughout the nation. The key to success is in combining appropriate methodology with well-qualified personnel and a comprehensive program of referral and follow-up.

Hearing screening of school-age children has been widely practiced since the 1930s. Some school-based programs include screening for OME. Age, developmental status, available instrumentation, screening personnel, and institutional resources, each of which will be considered in this chapter, determine the hearing screening method of choice. Screening newborn infants for middle ear effusion is not widely practiced because of difficulties with test interpretation; however, older infants, toddlers, and preschoolers are routinely screened for both hearing loss and OME.

VISUAL INSPECTION AND OTOSCOPY

Screening procedures begin with visual inspection of the external ear to detect noticeable signs of disease or malformation. The outer ear examination is followed by otoscopic inspection. The *otoscope*, an optical device that provides light and magnification, is used to examine the ear canal and tympanic membrane. Two common ways of holding the otoscope are illustrated in Figure 2–1. Either is acceptable as long as the child's head is supported to avoid injury or discomfort

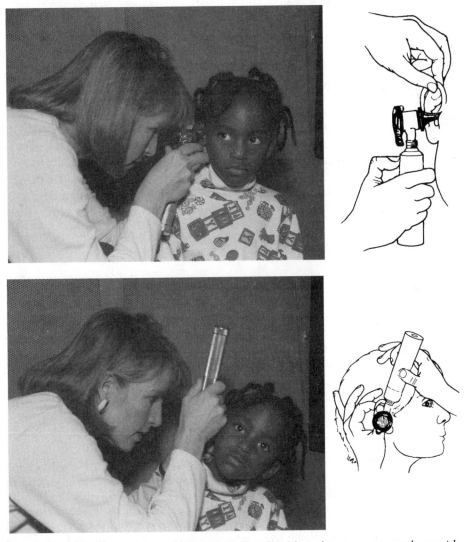

Figure 2-1   Two appropriate methods of holding the otoscope, each providing control of the child's head in the event of sudden movement. Line drawings adapted from Bluestone, Klein, and McKenna (1990), with permission.

in the event of sudden movement. Visual inspection is facilitated by gently pulling the pinna to straighten the ear canal, as illustrated in Figure 2–1. Some young children are fearful of the otoscope, so it is important to prepare the child before initiating the examination. Preparation is best accomplished by showing the instrument to the child and describing it as a "flashlight" for looking in the ear. With a reluctant child it is sometimes helpful to shine the light on his/her hand or to perform a quick otoscopic inspection on a doll or stuffed animal. Once the speculum is positioned in the child's ear canal the major landmarks of the tympanic membrane and middle ear can usually be seen. Figure 2–2 illustrates the principle landmarks partly visible through the translucent tympanic membrane. Note that the orientation of these structures changes from infancy to adulthood. Signs of external ear disease or canal occlusion (excess cerumen or a foreign object) should be noted and referred for medical management (Table 2–1). The presence of a tympanostomy tube should also be noted.

EXTERNAL AND OTOSCOPIC INSPECTION PROTOCOL

1. Carefully examine the external ear for signs of disease or malformation.
2. Show the otoscope to the child and briefly explain the procedure. Encourage the child to be still during the examination. A visual distraction device such as a video player can be helpful in gaining the child's cooperation.
3. Gently pull the pinna up and back while placing the speculum in the ear canal opening; carefully inspect the ear canal and tympanic membrane.
4. If the canal is unobstructed and there are no signs of ear disease, proceed

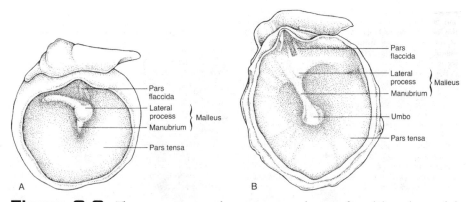

Figure 2-2 The tympanic membrane in a newborn infant (A) and an adult (B). Note that the infant tympanic membrane is almost horizontal. Lateral process of malleus is most prominent. Pars flaccida is thicker and more vascular. The adult's tympanic membrane is more vertical. Lateral process of malleus is less prominent. Manubrium of malleus is more vertical. Pars flaccida appears less vascular. (Adapted from Kenna, M. (1990), "Embryology and developmental anatomy of the ear." In Bluestone, C., & Stool, S., eds. *Pediatric Otolaryngology*, p. 79. Philadelphia: W. B. Saunders.)

TABLE 2-1 Conditions and diseases of the tympanic membrane and their treatment.

Disease or Condition	Description and Treatment
Tympanosclerosis	Thick white patches on the tympanic membrane resulting from deposits associated with previous ear disease or perforation. Usually there is little or no effect on hearing sensitivity; however, conductive hearing loss can occur if ossicles become embedded. Medical review is warranted but surgical intervention is rarely needed.
Retraction	A drawing inward of the tympanic membrane created by negative middle ear pressure. Treatment not indicated unless condition is chronic.
Myringitis	Inflammation of the tympanic membrane, usually associated with external otitis or otitis media. Requires medical referral; topical antibiotics are sometimes prescribed.
Perforation	An opening in the tympanic membrane usually caused by chronic otitis media but may be related to trauma or an extruded tympanostomy tube. Requires medical referral. Most perforations heal without treatment but some require surgical intervention.

with screening. If there is evidence of impacted cerumen, ear disease, or a foreign object, refer for medical management before proceeding further.

5. Discard disposable specula; put reusable specula in a disinfectant solution, out of reach of children.

OTOSCOPY PITFALLS AND PRACTICAL CONSIDERATIONS

- Be sure to select a speculum with a large enough diameter to facilitate visualization.
- Carefully place the speculum in the ear canal before bringing the eye to the viewing lens.
- Otoscopy must be completed prior to placement of probe tips or insert receivers because a foreign object in the ear canal could be dislodged by the probe, causing serious injury to the tympanic membrane and middle ear.

BEHAVIORAL METHODS OF HEARING ASSESSMENT

Pure Tone Threshold Audiometry

Pure tone *threshold* audiometry is designed to measure the lowest (softest) level a listener can detect when pure tone signals are presented via air or bone conduction. Hearing threshold testing is considered a diagnostic test, not a screening procedure, and therefore should be performed only by an audiologist or under the direct supervision of an audiologist. Pure tone threshold audiometry is reviewed here because of its importance in the description and classification of hearing loss. A modification of the behavioral pure tone threshold test known as "visual reinforcement audiometry" will also be described.

Routine *pure tone air conduction audiometry* involves the presentation of test stimuli from an audiometer (Figure 2–3). Testing is performed across a broad range of *frequencies* from low to high (250–8000 Hz) at octave intervals, and thresholds are plotted on an *audiogram* using the standard symbols shown in Figure 2–4. *Pure tone bone conduction audiometry* refers to the presentation of pure tone signals from a bone vibrator, placed behind the ear on the mastoid process (see Figure 2–5). *Bone conduction thresholds* are generally obtained only for the frequencies 250 through 4000 Hz, at octave intervals. Older children are instructed to raise their hand or press a response button when the tone is heard; younger children often respond by dropping a block or performing some other age-appropriate behavioral response. Conductive hearing loss is characterized by normal or near-normal bone conduction thresholds in the presence of abnormal (elevated) air conduction thresholds. When air and bone conduction thresholds are equal and abnormal, the loss is described as sensorineural (Figure 2–4). A mixed hearing loss is characterized by abnormal responses to air conduction and bone conduction, with air conduction thresholds poorer than bone conduction thresholds.

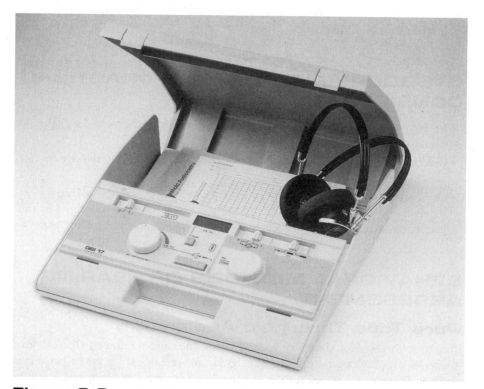

Figure 2-3 A portable pure tone audiometer with supra-aural earphones. Courtesy of Grason-Stadler.

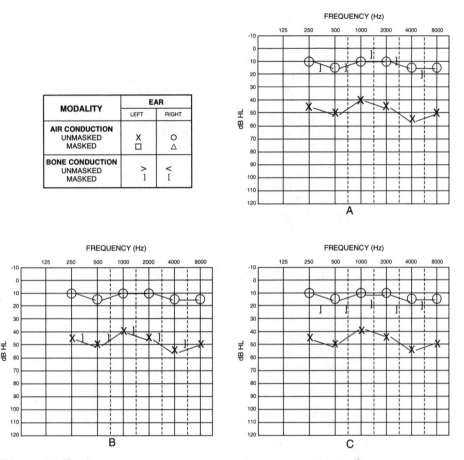

Figure 2-4 Audiograms illustrating a moderate unilateral *conductive* hearing loss, left ear (A), a moderate unilateral *sensorineural* hearing loss, left ear (B), and a moderate unilateral *mixed* hearing loss, left ear (C). In all three examples the right ear is within normal limits; masked bone conduction thresholds are shown for the left ear.

Although seemingly straightforward, pure tone threshold audiometry is often complicated by transmission of tones through the head from the test ear to the non-test ear. In order to isolate the test ear, the audiologist applies *masking noise* to the non-test ear. Masked threshold symbols are also shown in Figure 2–4.

Behavioral threshold assessment in the manner just described requires a developmental age of at least 2¹/₂ years. For infants and young toddlers in the age range from about 6 to 30 months, a modified threshold assessment procedure known as visual reinforcement audiometry (VRA) is used. Research has shown that test signals alone result in highly variable responses, but when the stimulus is paired with an interesting visual reinforcer (Figure 2–6), head-turn responses can be readily conditioned using basic operant conditioning procedures. In a typical VRA diagnostic evaluation performed by an audiologist, the infant is placed in a highchair or held by an adult, usually the parent (Figure 2–7). Test signals, which typically consist of frequency modulated (warbled)

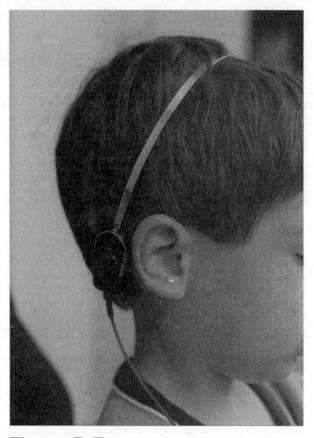

Figure 2-5 Bone conduction oscillator on the mastoid process of the temporal bone for pure tone testing.

pure tones, are presented from a loudspeaker in the corner of a sound-treated room. An assistant is seated across from the child to maintain attention away from the loudspeaker and reinforcer. The assessment begins when the audiologist, located outside the test room, presents a test stimulus. If the infant responds (head turn), the reinforcer is activated. The next stimulus is presented at a lower intensity level; if a response occurs, it is again reinforced. If there is no response the signal level is raised and another trial is conducted. A bracketing procedure is performed until a reliable estimate of hearing sensitivity is obtained. When test signals are delivered from a loudspeaker, the responses provide an indication of "better ear" sensitivity, as it cannot be determined which ear had better hearing sensitivity. Individual ear data can be obtained if the child will accept placement of insert receivers, described later in this chapter.

Unlike most of the screening procedures described in this text, VRA is conducted almost exclusively in audiology clinics. This is, in part, because of the need for specialized instrumentation including the reinforcement apparatus and calibrated test environment, where stimuli of known frequency and intensity can be delivered from loudspeakers. A properly calibrated environment usually

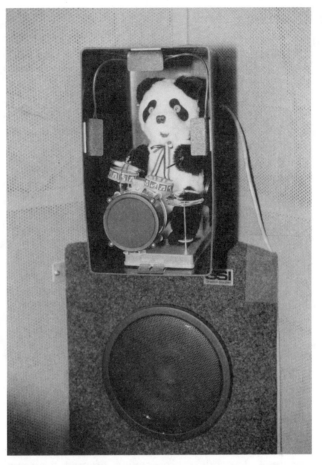

Figure 2-6 Reinforcement device used for conditioning a head-turn response in a young child during visual reinforcement audiometry. The plastic window has been removed to show the lights and moving toy.

requires a special sound-attenuated test room, or "sound suite," typically found only in an audiology clinic. Furthermore, behavioral assessment using VRA requires a considerable degree of clinical skill and experience. Indeed, behavioral assessment of children in this age range can be challenging even for an experienced clinician. For these reasons, ASHA screening guidelines recommend that VRA evaluations be conducted by an audiologist. Fortunately, the advent of otoacoustic emissions, described later in this chapter, provide a physiologic screening alternative to VRA that can be applied to this age group in more diverse settings, by non-audiology personnel.

There are many variations on the basic VRA paradigm. As noted earlier, individual ear data can be obtained when VRA is performed under earphones or with insert receivers. Multiple reinforcers can be used to maximize the child's interest and increase the number of responses. There are also variations in VRA

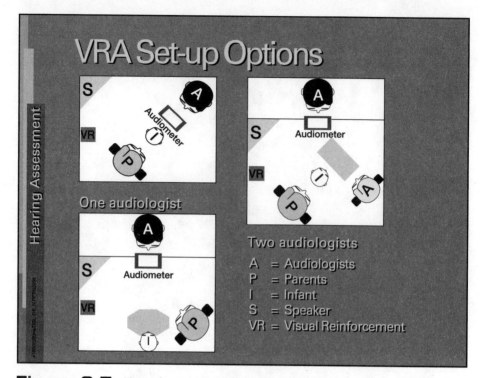

Figure 2-7 Typical set-ups for visual reinforcement audiometry (VRA) as performed by an audiologist in a calibrated sound suite. (Courtesy of Phonak)

assessment procedures. For example, some audiologists prefer to begin with ascending rather than descending presentation of pure tone stimuli. VRA can also be performed using computer-generated stimuli. Clinical protocols for VRA, as used in a hospital-based audiology clinic, are described in Chapter 7.

Pure Tone Screening

When the goal is to determine whether the listener can detect sounds at or above a certain fixed level of intensity, the procedure is described as *pure tone screening*. The screening level identifies a point separating those listeners whose hearing sensitivity is within normal limits from those with abnormal hearing. Pure tone screening is usually performed using air-conducted stimuli presented from an earphone or insert receiver (described shortly). For infants and toddlers at a developmental level of about 6–30 months, behavioral hearing screening can often be accomplished using "visual reinforcement audiometry" administered by an audiologist. For toddlers and preschool-age children, pure tone screening can be carried out using behavioral play techniques. Pure tone screening of cooperative children above the age of three years can generally be administered successfully by a variety of qualified health care providers and support personnel, with minimal time and equipment.

Pure Tone Screening with Play Audiometry

For children at a developmental level above three years of age, it is usually possible to accomplish behavioral pure tone screening with a portable audiometer using a procedure known as play audiometry (Figure 2–8 and Table 2–2). This usually takes the form of pure tone screening with signals presented at a fixed-intensity via earphones or insert receivers, so that each ear can be evaluated separately. The child responds by dropping a block in a container or participating in some other age-appropriate activity.

As illustrated in Figure 2–9, pure tones may be presented from standard earphones or insert receivers. Each method of delivery has advantages and disadvantages. The standard audiometric headset shown in Figure 2–9A has been in use for many years. Advantages include ease of placement and durability. Because of their size and weight, however, they may not be accepted as readily by young children. Insert receivers (Figure 2–9B), which are placed in the ear canal and secured by foam cushions, are often better tolerated by young children because nothing is worn on or over the head. Recall that insert receivers are also advantageous because they provide greater reduction of background noise. Since they are placed within the ear canal, however, the foam cushions should be replaced for each child, thus increasing the time and cost of each individual screening. Insert receivers have important advantages when used by the audiologist for clinical testing, but for routine screening in a suitable acoustic environment, standard audiometric earphones are more convenient. Regardless

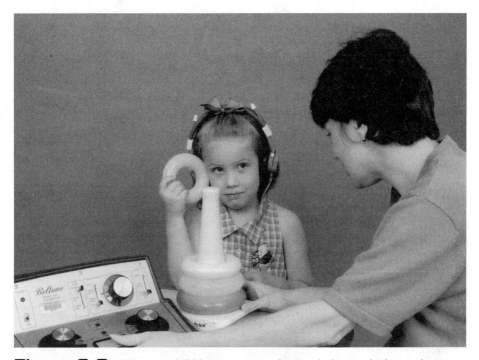

Figure 2-8 A young child being screened using behavioral play audiometry. Note placement of the audiometer to prevent visual cues.

TABLE 2-2	Standard features of a portable pure-tone audiometer.
Audiometer	**Description and Purpose**
Power source	Most portable audiometers have a power cord designed to operate from a standard electrical outlet. When selecting a screening site it is important to consider availability of a power source. If an extension cord is needed, wires must be safely situated. Duct tape or rubber strips designed for this purpose can be employed where hazards exist.
Power switch	All audiometers have an on/off switch. The switch should be in the "off" position when the power supply is connected or disconnected.
Frequency selector	Most portable audiometers produce air conducted pure tones ranging from 250 to 8000 Hz. For screening purposes, the recommended frequencies are 1000, 2000, and 4000 Hz.
Attenuator dial	The attenuator dial determines the output level of the test tone. The attenuator dial typically covers a range from 0 to 110 dB HL in 5 dB steps. For screening purposes, the recommended output level is 20 dB HL.
Earphones and insert receivers	Standard supra-aural earphones and insert receivers have advantages and disadvantages (see text).The red earphone (or insert receiver) is used for the right ear and the blue earphone (or insert receiver) is used with the left ear. Earphones and insert receivers are not interchangeable among audiometers; each pair is calibrated to a specific audiometer.
Output selector	Audiometers have a dial or switch that directs the tone to either the right or left earphone. Earphones/insert receivers must be correctly routed so that the output selector corresponds to the appropriate right/left transducer.

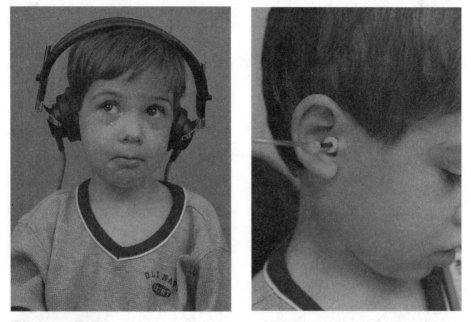

Figure 2-9 Supra-aural earphones (A) and insert receiver (B) for delivery of air conducted pure tone signals.

of whether earphones or insert receivers are used, it is important to note that they are not interchangeable among audiometers; that is, each is calibrated for use with a specific audiometer.

Personnel for Pure Tone Screening

Institutional hearing screening programs should be performed under the general supervision of an audiologist; however, the actual screening procedures may be carried out by a speech-language pathologist, nurse, or qualified support personnel. Children screened on an individual basis, for example in a pediatrician's office, will often be seen by a nurse or nurse assistant. The screening procedures, as described below, are not difficult; however, they require good rapport with children and careful attention to the proper use of the audiometer. Inexperienced personnel should obtain inservice orientation by an audiologist, followed by hands-on experience with cooperative children. State licensure laws and regulations should always be consulted with respect to screening personnel. In many states, only audiologists, licensed hearing aid dispensers, or personnel employed in a medical setting can obtain thresholds measures. In contrast, a broad range of health care providers and qualified support personnel can conduct pure tone *screening* of preschool and school-age children.

The Pure Tone Screening Environment

The test environment must be carefully selected since a valid pure tone hearing screening cannot be conducted in an environment with high levels of competing background noise. Table 2–3 provides a summary of permissible noise levels, according to American National Standards Institute (ANSI) standards. The values shown are sound pressure levels for "octave bands" around the frequencies of interest. Ambient (background) noise levels must be at or below the sound levels indicated in the table. Generally these measurements are made by an audiologist or acoustic engineer using a sound level meter; however, other personnel, if properly trained and equipped, can also measure ambient noise levels.

Ideally, all screening environments will be in full compliance with guidelines for acceptable ambient noise levels. Unfortunately, two practical problems often occur. First, the equipment and personnel needed to accomplish sound level measurements may be unavailable. Second, even if the necessary resources are available, it is unlikely that ambient levels will remain constant over time.

TABLE 2–3 Maximum permissible ambient noise levels in dB SPL for screening at 20 dB HL at the frequencies 1000, 2000, and 4000 Hz. ANSI S3.1–1991. These values represent dB levels for third-octave bands at the screening frequency, measured with a sound level meter.

	Frequency in Hz		
Condition	1000	2000	4000
Screening at 20 dB HL with supra-aural earphones	46.5	48.0	54.5
Screening at 20 dB HL with insert earphones	67.5	61.5	69.5

When sound level measurements are unavailable or when levels fluctuate, the examiner must use his or her judgment to determine the adequacy of the acoustic environment.

When the screening environment is less than ideal, it is often tempting to increase the presentation level (dB HL) in a noisy environment. This temptation must be avoided at all times. Locating a suitable test environment requires planning and perseverance, but most institutional settings have a few places quiet enough to conduct valid hearing screening. In an elementary school, the library can often be used if scheduled in advance. In a preschool, an office or health room can sometimes be used. When confronted with a questionable ambient noise situation, careful listening checks and sound level measurements are needed. Those responsible for financing the screening program must understand the importance of an adequate acoustic environment. Indeed, costs will be far higher in the long run if children are unnecessarily referred for additional testing because of unsuitable screening conditions. Similarly, increasing the tone to a higher intensity level in order to "compensate" for a poor acoustic environment could result in an even more costly error: failure to identify a child with a hearing loss. Additional information regarding the pure tone-screening environment is provided in Chapter 8.

Calibration of Pure Tone Audiometers

Audiometers must undergo complete calibration checks by a qualified technician at least once each year. The importance of calibration cannot be overstated! The American National Standards Institute (ANSI) has established formal guidelines and procedures for calibrating audiometric instruments. Suppliers of audiometric equipment usually provide calibration services or they can make a referral to a qualified technician. In addition to formal calibration checks, ANSI standards also advise daily listening checks. A protocol for daily listening checks is presented in Table 2–4. It is important to follow these procedures faithfully before and during a screening program.

TABLE 2-4 Protocol for daily listening checks and audiometer inspection.	
Visual inspection	• Power cord: Good condition with solid connections at each end; three-prong plug.
	• Earphone cords: Good condition with solid connections at each earphone and with plugs fully inserted in the appropriate jack.
	• Earphone cushions: Clean and flexible.
	• Control panel: Dials/switches clean and properly aligned.
Listening check	• After a 10-minute warm-up period, place earphones/insert receivers as they will be used during screening, and listen carefully.
	• Present tones at each screening frequency, at several different output levels. While listening, move the cords. There should be steady output with no clicks, static, or other noises.

When to Perform Pure Tone Screening

All children should be screened at least once in the preschool years and again at entry to elementary school. As universal hearing screening programs expand across the nation, identification is occurring at an earlier age. Nevertheless, hearing screening should be provided any time parents or caretakers have concerns about hearing, even if the child has previously passed a hearing screening. There could be a late onset sensorineural hearing loss or, more commonly, a transient conductive loss associated with otitis media. It is also possible that the previous hearing screening was, for some reason, invalid. In any event, concerns of parents or caretakers should always be followed up with a hearing screening or referral to an audiologist, depending on the child's age and developmental status.

For preschool-aged children, the time of year chosen to perform group hearing screening is an important consideration. Although hearing screening can be provided at any time, there are advantages to conducting this activity in the fall of the year. For children in preschool or elementary grades, fall marks the beginning of a new school year. It is obviously desirable to identify hearing problems early in the school year so that appropriate intervention can be undertaken. The fall and winter months are also associated with a higher incidence of otitis media. Although this is not true in all regions, more children with transient hearing and middle ear problems are likely to be identified during this time of year. The time of day is also important. Preschoolers generally perform best from mid to late morning. Timing is less critical once children reach school age. In older children, instructional schedules are likely to dictate when screening can be conducted.

In summary, hearing screening for children should be provided: 1) at least once during the preschool years, preferably at birth as part of a universal hearing screening program; 2) upon school entry; 3) periodically during the school years; 4) any time parents or caretakers suspect a hearing loss; and 5) yearly for children receiving special services or for children needing surveillance because of a condition that increases the risk of delayed-onset hearing loss (see Table 1–6).

Interpretation of Pure Tone Screening Results

In order to pass, the child must respond at least twice at every screening frequency in each ear. If the child does not respond it may simply be due to lack of cooperation or motivation; however, hearing loss should always be suspected until it can be appropriately ruled out. If there is a hearing loss, the underlying nature of the loss (conductive vs. sensorineural) cannot be determined from pure tone screening, as bone conduction testing is required to make this determination. Thus, children who do not pass the hearing screening should be referred to an audiologist for a complete assessment.

Target Populations for Pure Tone Screening

Pure tone screening using behavioral play techniques can be successfully applied to most children at a developmental level of approximately three years. Pure tone screening is *not* recommended:

• When the screening environment is excessively noisy;

- When the child cannot be reliably conditioned (this will include most children under the age of three years).

Screening Protocol for Play Audiometry

1. Perform otoscopic inspection of each external ear and ear canal. In the event of complete occlusion (impacted cerumen), foreign object, or visible signs of ear disease, refer for medical management before proceeding.
2. Seat the child in a chair next to the table with a portable audiometer. Explain what the child will hear and how he/she is to respond: "You will hear some beeps in the earphone; whenever you hear one, even if it's very soft, <examiner demonstrates the response>. "Be sure to wait until you hear it. Listen carefully."
3. Place the earphones or insert receivers (red phone, right ear; blue phone, left ear) and demonstrate the appropriate response by presenting a tone assumed to be audible (e.g., 1000 Hz at 40 dB HL), and then assist the child with the desired response. If the child does not respond at 40 dB HL, rescreen later or refer for audiologic assessment. If the child performs the task independently, explain that the tones will become very soft and may be heard in either ear.
4. Set the attenuator to 20 dB HL and present the tone. Obtain at least two responses at each of the screening frequencies: 1000 Hz, 2000 Hz, and 4000 Hz.
5. Interpret and record screening results. In order to pass the child must respond to at least two test presentations at all test frequencies in each ear.
6. Arrange for referral or follow-up, as needed.

Play Audiometry Pitfalls and Practical Considerations

- The examiner must be careful to avoid visual cues when presenting the test stimulus. Subtle movement of the arm, hand, or eyes, for example, can invalidate the test.
- Whenever possible, select a site relatively free of visual distractions.
- The examiner must be certain that the earphones are comfortably adjusted to fit directly over (earphones) or in the ear (insert receivers) with the red earphone on the right ear and the blue earphone on the left ear. When possible it is best to direct the cords behind rather than in front of the child.
- It is important to make sure the child understands exactly what is expected before starting the test. A few extra minutes with orientation and demonstration can save considerable time and expense in the long run by reducing unnecessary referrals for rescreening.
- Be certain that earphones are adjusted carefully so that they fit snugly against the ear canal opening. If using insert receivers, they must be carefully shaped and fully inserted into the canal opening.

Speech Stimuli for Hearing Screening

Because young children generally respond more readily to speech than to tonal stimuli, it is logical to consider speech as a method of screening for hearing loss. Unfortunately, speech is not well suited for this purpose. The spectral characteristics of speech are such that hard-of-hearing children are often able to identify a word or picture based on minimal acoustic cues. The child whose audiogram

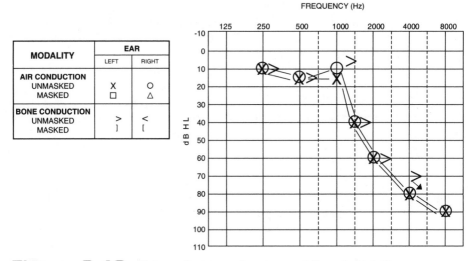

Figure 2-10 This audiogram, showing a bilateral high-frequency sensorineural hearing loss, illustrates the importance of using frequency-specific stimuli (pure tones) for hearing screening. This child erroneously "passed" a hearing screening based on normal thresholds for speech stimuli.

appears in Figure 2–10 erroneously "passed" a hearing screening because he responded well to speech stimuli based on his normal hearing sensitivity in the low frequencies (pure tone screening was not performed). Obviously, children with substantial hearing loss can be missed when screening is based on speech signals alone. Thus, pure tone screening, administered on an individual basis with a portable audiometer, remains the behavioral hearing screening method of choice for most children at a developmental level above three years of age.

PHYSIOLOGIC METHODS OF SCREENING FOR HEARING LOSS

Physiologic tests of auditory function, which include otoacoustic emissions and auditory brainstem responses, are not direct measures of hearing. Rather, they are tests that allow the clinician to make inferences regarding a child's hearing based on physiologic measures. They are considered objective because they do not involve the active participation of the child or the interpretation of the child's behavior. They do, however, require the child's general cooperation to the extent that probe or electrode placement is tolerated. Sometimes it is necessary to conduct these tests while the child is in natural sleep or under sedation.

Otoacoustic Emissions

In the 1970s it was discovered that the normal, healthy inner ear emits low-intensity sounds that can be detected by a sensitive microphone placed in the ear canal. These low-intensity sounds are called *otoacoustic emissions* (OAEs). Some ears have measurable OAEs even in the absence of auditory stimulation (spontaneous OAEs) but nearly every ear with normal middle ear and cochlear function will produce measurable OAEs in response to auditory stimulation.

Research has shown that OAEs originate in the outer hair cells through a process that allows the hair cells to act on signals as they reach the cochlea. This process results in a replication or "echo" of the incoming signals generated within the cochlea. Successful recording of OAEs not only requires a healthy cochlea but also necessitates normal or near-normal middle ear function. This is because OAE measurement relies on the middle ear conductive mechanism (tympanic membrane and ossicles) first to transmit the stimuli to the inner ear and then to convey the cochlear emissions, by way of reverse transmission, back into the ear canal where recording takes place. OAEs are said to be "preneural" because they occur only at the level of the cochlea, thus permitting sensory function to be evaluated apart from higher level processing. OAEs are ideally suited for hearing screening because sensory hearing loss invariably affects cochlear function.

When OAEs are elicited by an acoustic stimulus they are said to be "evoked." The acoustic stimuli most commonly used are "clicks" or pairs of tones. Click-evoked emissions produce *transient evoked otoacoustic emissions* (TEOAEs) while emissions evoked by tone pairs produce *distortion product otoacoustic emissions* (DPOAEs). Each will be considered separately.

Transient evoked otoacoustic emissions (TEOAEs) are generated in response to brief acoustic click stimuli. In a typical TEOAE evaluation, a series of clicks, each with a duration of approximately 100 microseconds (μsec), is delivered through a probe assembly in the ear canal using instrumentation depicted in Figure 2–11. The probe contains a miniature microphone for recording the OAE responses that normally occur 4–10 μsec following stimulation. Before they can be viewed and analyzed, the responses must be amplified, filtered, and digitized by a computer. The resulting waveform is said to be frequency-specific because the shorter-latency high frequencies emerge first, followed by the longer-latency low frequencies. Recall from Chapter 1 that this follows the coding pattern of the basilar membrane in the cochlea. It is now known that the cochlear hair cells play an important role in fine-tuning the basilar membrane's vibration pattern. The separation of the TEOAE from other recorded noise is accomplished by correlating pairs of recorded responses: the higher the correlation, the more the recorded response is assumed to be dominated by the OAE. These analyses allow the TEOAE to be expressed in terms of "signal-to-noise ratios" for various frequency bands. A signal-to-noise ratio of 6 dB, that is, a

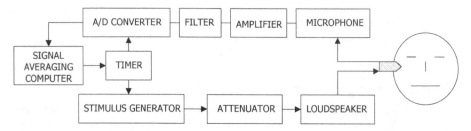

Figure 2-11 Block diagram of instrumentation for recording transient evoked otoacoustic emissions (TEOAEs).

response that emerges from the noise by at least 6 dB; is usually required to verify the presence of a TEOAE response in a given frequency band (see Figure 2–12).

When there is damage anywhere along the basilar membrane, OAEs will be absent for that frequency region. Although there is not an exact correspondence between audiometric thresholds and TEOAEs, emissions will be absent or abnormal when there is cochlear hearing loss greater than 30–40 dB.

In general, TEOAEs diminish with increasing age even if hearing sensitivity remains normal. Fortunately, TEOAEs are especially robust in newborn infants, but middle ear fluid and debris remaining from the birth process, including vernix in the ear canal, may complicate the recording of TEOAEs in newborn infants. Even so, programs with experienced personnel report reasonable success with TEOAE in newborn screening, as evidenced by pass rates exceeding 90%. A newborn infant undergoing TEOAE evaluation is shown in Figure 2–13.

Stimulus and recording parameters vary based on the target population, the goals of the screening program, and the instrumentation employed. ASHA screening guidelines (1997) recommend that TEOAEs be recorded using broadband clicks presented at a rate of 50–80 per second at 80 dB SPL. Automated instruments, which are now used almost exclusively for screening purposes, have pre-selected stimulus and recording parameters.

Distortion product otoacoustic emissions (DPOAEs) arise from the simultaneous presentation of two tones via a probe assembly in the subject's ear canal. The two tones interact in the cochlea to generate a third (distortion) tone, produced by the outer hair cells of the healthy cochlea. The two stimulus tones are called *primaries* and the third tone is the distortion product. The frequency of the distortion product can be predicted based on the frequency relationship of the two primaries. Specifically, the third tone will occur at a frequency equal to two times the frequency of the first primary minus that of the second, or, $2f1–f2$. For example, as depicted in Figure 2–14, simultaneously presented stimulus tones at $f1 = 3264$ Hz and $f2 = 3928$ Hz would produce a distortion product at 2600 Hz ($6528 - 3828 = 2500$).

Instrumentation depicted in Figure 2–15 is used to generate and analyze the responses. Criteria for the presence of a DPOAE include a comparison of the level at the expected DPOAE frequency to the noise levels in the surrounding frequency regions; this provides a measure of signal-to-noise ratio. As with TEOAEs, a signal-to-noise ratio of at least 6 dB is usually considered a minimum for the verification of a DPOAE.

When DPOAEs are used for hearing screening, the frequency ratio of the two tones and their respective presentation levels have a significant effect on the resulting DPOAEs. Although there is no universal standard, a frequency ratio of 1.22 (e.g., 1000 Hz and 1220 Hz) appears to produce the largest DPOAEs. Another important consideration is the presentation level (dB) of the primary tones. When DPOAEs are used for screening, they usually involve "unequal primaries," that is, different presentation levels for the two primary tones. Thus, screening protocols typically require a lower stimulus level for the higher frequency primary (L2) than that of the lower frequency (L1) primary. For example, an L2 stimulus level 10–15 dB lower than the L1 stimulus level is often used. When distortion products are evoked across a range of frequencies, it is

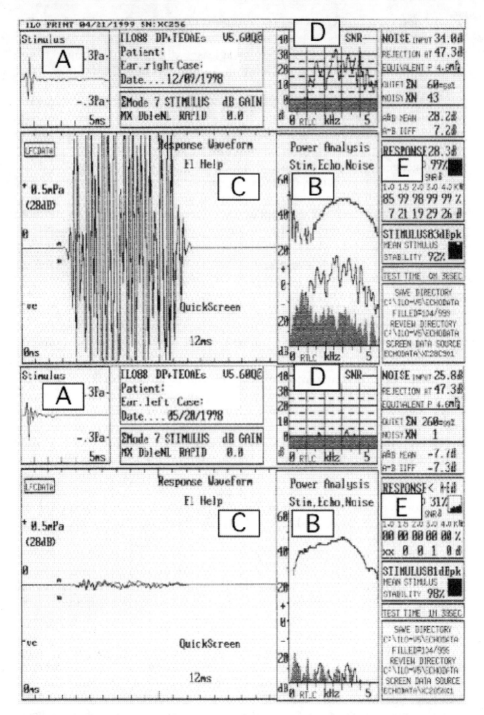

Figure 2-12 Sample recordings from two newborn infants, one with present TEOAEs (upper half of figure) and the other with absent TEOAEs (lower half of figure). Panel A: time waveform of click stimulus. Panel B: spectrum of click stimulus (upper solid line), TEOAE (lower solid line), and noise floor (shaded area). Panel C: time waveform of TEOAE. Panel D: normalized spectrum of TEOAE. Panel E: signal-to-noise ratios within defined frequency bands of the response. From Roush and Grose (in press).

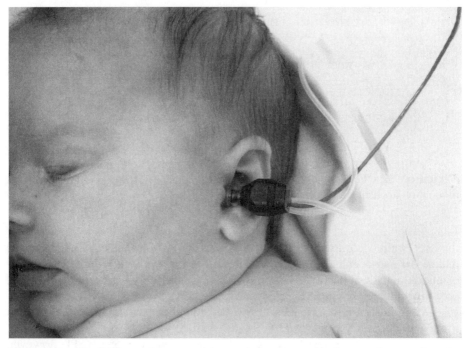

Figure 2-13 Probe assembly in the ear canal of a newborn infant for recording of otoacoustic emissions (OAEs).

possible to construct a "DPgram." The DPgram is a plot of 2f1–f2 distortion products as a function of the f2 frequency regions (or geometric mean of f1 and f2).

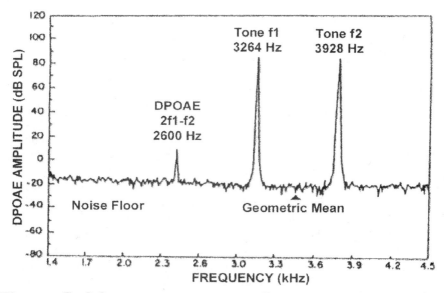

Figure 2-14 Illustration of DPOAE at 2600 Hz generated by the simultaneous presentation of tones at 3264 Hz (F1) and 3928 Hz (F2).

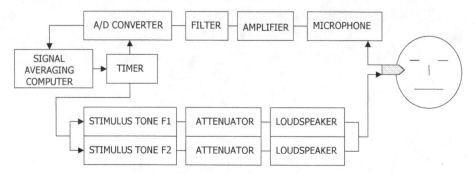

Figure 2-15 Block diagram of instrumentation for recording distortion product otoacoustic emissions (DPOAEs).

As with TEOAEs, DPOAEs are generally present in ears with normal middle ear and cochlear function, and absent in ears with outer hair cell damage or middle ear dysfunction. Examples of normal and abnormal DPOAEs plotted on a DPgram are shown in Figures 2–16 and 2–17.

ASHA screening guidelines (1997) recommend that DPOAEs be recorded using the frequency ratio of f2/f1 = 1.2 with f2 at 2000, 3000 and 4000 Hz. Suggested presentation levels are L2 = 55 dB SPL and L1 = 65 dB SPL; however, as with TEOAEs, most automated instruments designed for screening purposes have pre-selected stimulus and recording parameters (see Table 2–5).

Automated OAE Recording

Automated instruments for OAE screening are available from several different manufacturers. Most of the instruments designed for automated OAE recording simply indicate "pass" or "refer." Even so, examiners must be skilled in using the device selected and well informed regarding the interpretation of screening results. Comprehensive inservice education by an audiologist is needed for all screening personnel.

Interpretation of OAEs

OAEs are ideally suited for screening purposes. Recall, however, that OAEs will be absent if there is a significant middle ear problem. This is an important consideration as the populations often targeted for hearing screening—infants and young children—may have conductive hearing loss caused by OME. Newborns are unlikely to have OME, but there may be vernix in the ear canal and residual amniotic fluid or other debris in the middle ear. When these conditions result in a conductive hearing loss, reverse transmission of the OAE (from the cochlea back to the ear canal) is reduced and in some cases eliminated. When OAEs *are* recorded, whether by TEOAE or DPOAE, the findings are an indication of normal hearing or no more than a mild hearing loss. Absent OAEs, on the other hand, may be due to a variety of conditions ranging from conductive hearing loss associated with OME to profound sensorineural hearing loss. It is important to emphasize that OAEs cannot be used to determine the type or degree of hearing loss. Infants who do not pass an OAE screening should be referred to an

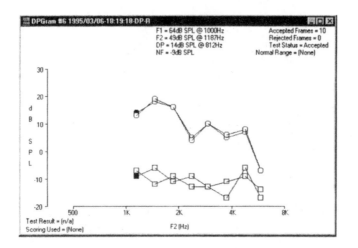

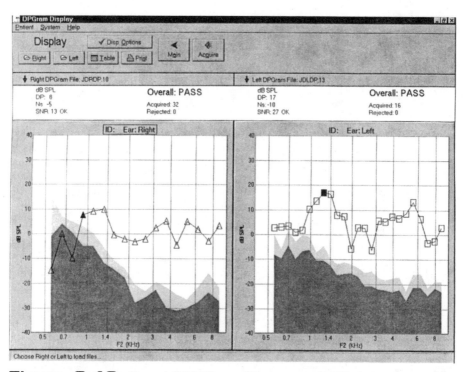

Figure 2-16 Normal DPOAEs as they appear on DPgrams generated by two commercially available instruments. In the top panel, the levels of the DPOAEs (open circles) are plotted as a function of the upper primary tone (F2); the squares indicate the noise floor. Note good replicability of two consecutive tests on the same ear. In the lower panel, triangles and squares (right and left ears) represent the levels of the DPOAEs; the shaded area indicates noise floor.

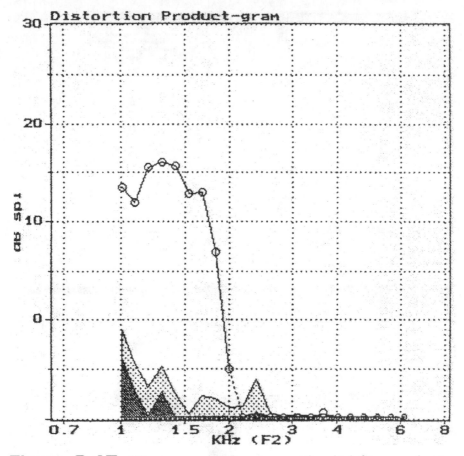

Figure 2-17 DPgram recorded for an ear with a high-frequency hearing loss. The levels of the DPOAE (open circles) are plotted as a function of the upper primary tone (F2); lower hatched area indicates noise floor.

audiologist for assessment. In some programs, rescreening occurs in the hospital prior to discharge. A program model that employs OAEs in the newborn nursery is presented in Chapter 6.

In rare cases OAEs may be present indicating normal outer-hair cell function (consistent with normal hearing) while inner hair cell or neural function may be abnormal. A condition described as *auditory neuropathy* (see Chapter 1) may occur, especially in infants with histories of hyperbilirubinemia or other illness requiring neonatal intensive care. It is important to note that OAE screening will not identify infants with auditory neuropathy.

When and Where to Perform OAE Screening

OAE screening can be performed as part of an institutional screening protocol or on an individual basis when there are parent or caretaker concerns regarding the child's hearing. When used in the newborn nursery, most programs obtain OAE measures prior to discharge because of the difficulties often encountered with

TABLE 2-5 Pass/refer criteria for several DPOAE screeners.	
DPOAE system	**Pass/fail criteria**
Biologic AuDX	*DPMin:* −7, −8, −5, −6 dB SPL at 2k, 3k, 4k, and 5kHz, respectively *MinSNR:* 6 dB at all test frequencies *Overall Test Pass:* 3/4 test frequencies must meet above criteria Customizable on AuDXII and AuDXPlus
Etymotic Research ERO-SCAN	*DPMin:* −5 dB SPL at 2k, 3k, and 4kHZ *MinSNR:* 5 dB at all test frequencies *Overall Test Pass:* 3/3 test frequencies must meet above criteria Customizable
Grason-Stadler GSI-70	*DPMin:* −3, −3, −5 dB SPL at 2k, 3k, and 4kHz, respectively *MinSNR:* 10 dB at all test frequencies *Overall Test Pass:* 3/3 test frequencies have to meet above criteria Customizable on GSI70 Multiple Patient Version
Intelligent Hearing Systems SmartOAE	No default pass/refer criterion
Starkey DP2000	No default pass/refer criterion
Sonamed Clarity System	*DPMin:* −5 dB SPL from 2000–5000 Hz *MinSNR:* 5 dB from 2000–5000 Hz *MaxNF:* 10(1–2K), 5(2–4K), 0(4–8K) *Replicability* (dB separation) = 3 *Overall Test Pass:* User specifiable Customizable
Madsen-Celesta	No default pass/refer criterion *DPMin:* Distortion product minimum amplitude *MinSNR:* Minimum signal-to-noise ratio *MaxNF:* Maximum allowable noise floor

follow-up and scheduling of return visits; however, programs vary in how and when they inform parents of screening results, as noted in Part II of this text.

When OAE screening is performed with toddlers and preschoolers it is usually conducted at child-care facilities. Screening usually takes place in the fall of the year and results are sent home via written communication. Part II of this text provides further discussion and additional information regarding communication with families.

Target Populations for OAE Screening

In recent years, OAEs have been used primarily with neonates and infants. Portable, automated instruments are now being used successfully in hundreds of hospitals. OAEs can also be applied to preschool and school-age children (see Figure 2–18). Since OAEs are affected by both sensory (cochlear) dysfunction and conductive (middle ear) disorders, they may be an ideal first-level screen for detection of hearing loss *and* otitis media. Several pilot studies have demonstrated

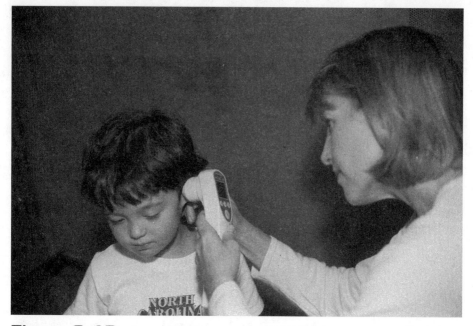

Figure 2-18 A portable battery-operated DPOAE instrument used to screen a preschool age child.

the potential utility of OAEs for such applications but larger-scale investigations have only recently been undertaken. Because of their convenience as well as their sensitivity to both middle and inner ear disease, it is anticipated that OAEs will play an ever-expanding role in the identification of hearing loss and otitis media across all age groups. At this time, OAE screening is widely used in a variety of settings:

- Newborn infants in a well-baby nursery (i.e., universal infant hearing screening).
- High-risk infants in a special care nursery.
- High-risk infants not previously screened for hearing loss.
- Children whose developmental level and/or physical limitations preclude behavioral hearing screening.

OAE screening is *not* recommended:

- When there are signs or symptoms of acute otitis media or other ear disease.
- When otoscopic inspection reveals impacted cerumen or a foreign object.
- When excessive movement or lack of cooperation precludes valid assessment.
- When the goals of the screening program include identification of auditory neuropathy.

Personnel for OAE Screening

Professionals and support personnel from many disciplines are now using OAEs. Nurses are often responsible for OAE screening of newborns. In other settings, speech pathologists, pediatricians, and support personnel have successfully used OAEs. Although OAE recording with automated instruments is relatively uncomplicated, the overall administration of the screening program requires careful management of numerous technical, personnel, and inter-institutional communications related to referral and follow-up. For this reason it is strongly recommended that institutional screening programs be conducted under the general supervision of an audiologist. It is also important to determine that personnel engaged in OAE screening operate in a manner consistent with state licensure, professional scope of practice, and other regulatory requirements. OAE technology is ideally suited for screening children on an individual basis, for example, in a pediatrician's office. In settings where an audiologist is not directly involved, it is important for screening personnel to have the information needed for audiologic referral when test results indicate the need for further evaluation.

Test Environment for OAE Screening

Measurement of OAEs requires a relatively quiet environment in a site where equipment does not interfere with other activities. Many hospital nurseries have procedure rooms ideally suited for this activity. Since healthy newborns spend a considerable amount of time in the mother's room, testing at maternal bedside has also been attempted. Unfortunately, this approach has had limited success because of fluctuating noise levels and other disturbances. In general, newborns are most efficiently screened in a quiet room within the newborn nursery.

When OAE testing is performed in schools and preschools it is often possible, with advance planning, to use a health room, library, or media center. The portability of modern OAE instruments allows considerable flexibility in how and when screening is performed.

Screening Protocol for OAE

1. Perform otoscopic inspection of each ear and ear canal. In the event of complete occlusion (impacted cerumen), foreign object, or visible signs of ear disease, refer for medical management before proceeding.
2. For older children, explain what will occur: "I'm going to put this soft tip in your ear (show probe tip and assembly). You will hear some sounds but all you need to do is hold still while the machine makes a picture with your ear. Be sure to hold still so we get a good picture . . ."
3. Place the probe in the child's ear and obtain the OAE measures.
4. Record and interpret the screening results. Automated OAE systems use a variety of "pass" criteria (see Table 2–5); a signal-to-noise ratio of at least 6 dB is usually required.
5. Arrange for referral/follow-up, as needed.

Referral and Follow-Up

Children suspected of hearing loss based on OAEs should be referred to an audiologist. Some programs perform rescreening prior to referral. Careful consideration must be given to how and when parents are informed of the screening results. See Parts II and III of this text for further discussion of communicating test results to family members.

OAE Pitfalls and Practical Considerations

- Room noise must be minimized to the extent possible.
- Infants who are bathed, fed, and sleepy tend to require the shortest test times.
- The probe tip should allow a snug fit in the ear canal.
- The probe tip must be firmly but carefully inserted to ensure stability during the test.
- The probe port must be carefully inspected before each test to make sure it is not occluded by cerumen or other debris. If occluded, the operator's manual should be consulted for proper cleaning.
- The microphone cable should be situated to avoid rubbing against moving surfaces (e.g., movements generated by the baby's breathing) that generate noise in the ear canal.
- When screening newborns, gentle massaging of external ear prior to insertion of the probe tip may improve recording.

Auditory Brainstem Responses

Auditory evoked potentials are physiologic responses recorded from electrodes attached to the head, in response to auditory stimuli presented from an insert receiver. These electrical events are classified according to their *post-stimulus latency*, or the amount of time that elapses from the onset of the stimulus to the appearance of the waveform. The earliest responses, 0–10 msec, reflect electrical activity of the VIIIth (auditory) nerve and brainstem and are described collectively as *auditory brainstem responses* (ABRs). "Middle latency" evoked potentials occur from about 10 msec to 100 msec and are believed to reflect sensory areas of the midbrain and auditory cortex. Late responses (70–300 msec and beyond) originate from the auditory cortex. The middle and late components are sometimes useful in evaluating higher level auditory processing but are not routinely used for screening. In contrast, the ABR (0–10 msec) has great utility for screening purposes.

The instrumentation used to record the ABR controls the timing and presentation of stimuli (typically 100 μsec clicks) and the recording of electrical activity generated within the auditory nerve and brainstem (see Figure 2–19). Amplification and signal averaging allow the electrical events time-locked with the stimulus to be differentiated from randomly distributed noise generated within the body and from external sources. With repeated sampling, the ABR emerges as a series of peaks, each associated with different neural generators

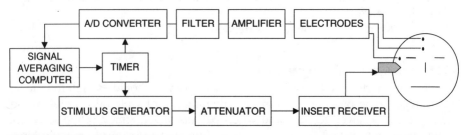

Figure 2-19 Block diagram of instrumentation used to record auditory brainstem responses.

within the auditory system (Figure 2–20). Waves I and II are produced by the auditory nerve. Waves III through V originate in proximal regions of the auditory nerve through various levels of the auditory brainstem from the cochlear nucleus to the lateral lemniscus (see Chapter 1). ABRs are well suited for clinical use because they are minimally affected by the child's state of arousal. For example, audiologists measure ABR thresholds in sleeping or sedated infants. When recording conditions are optimal, wave V, the largest component, can be observed at levels close to the behavioral threshold.

As illustrated in Figure 2–20, the ABR changes as a function of age. Wave I latency in normal infants is mature at about 3 months of age, but waves III and V do not reach adult latency values until about 18 months. Consequently, the latency between waves (inter-wave latency) also changes with age. For example, the normal adult interwave interval (waves I–V) is approximately 4.0 msec to 4.5 msec, but the normal newborn interwave latency is about 5.0 msec. The appearance of the waveforms (also known as waveform morphology) is also affected by age. Typical infant ABR waveforms are shown in comparison to a typical adult waveform in Figure 2–20. Note the changes in waveform morphology as well as latency. Using clicks in combination with frequency-specific stimuli presented by air conduction and bone conduction, the audiologist uses diagnostic ABR testing to estimate the nature and degree of hearing loss. Figure 2–21 illustrates ABR recordings from a child with one normal ear and one unresponsive ear.

It is important to emphasize that the ABR is not a test of hearing in the perceptual sense. Rather, it is a test that provides information regarding the functional integrity of the auditory nerve and auditory regions of the brainstem. Normal timing and synchrony of neural firing from the auditory nerve through the auditory brainstem must occur in order to record the ABR. When the ABR appears at high levels of stimulation but is absent at levels within the range of normal hearing sensitivity, the results can be attributed to cochlear damage. Thus, the ABR can serve as a physiologic alternative to behavioral measures of hearing sensitivity.

Automated ABR

ABR screening is performed using automated instruments. Automated auditory brainstem response (AABR) testing is based on responses obtained from preselected stimulus and recording parameters. Instead of displaying waveforms requiring interpretation, the results are simply reported as pass or refer. For example, the AABR instrument shown in Figure 2–22, which has been in widespread use for many years, screens at a level of 35 dBnHL. Most AABR instruments are designed to compare the acquired ABR to normal ABR responses stored in computer memory. Specifically, the acquired response is compared to a stored template and expressed according to how well it matches the template, based on a statistical test known as the likelihood ratio. In order to generate a "pass," the criterion provides a level of confidence exceeding 99.9% that a response is present. Automated instruments for AABR vary in the way screening outcomes are reported so the operator must be thoroughly familiar with the instrument used. Fortunately, the ease of operation afforded by AABR instruments allows them to be used by nurses, support personnel, and others. A program model that employs AABRs in the newborn nursery is summarized in Chapter 5.

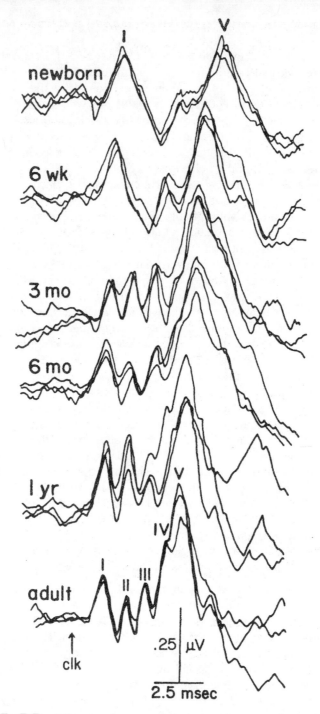

Figure 2-20 ABR waveforms recorded at various ages from a normal infant and from an adult. Note slight decrease in wave I latency and marked decrease in latency of waves III and V. Waves II, III, and IV become more distinct by the third month after birth. Adapted from Musiek & Rintelmann, *Contemporary perspectives in hearing assessment* (1999). Boston: Allyn & Bacon. Reprinted with permission.

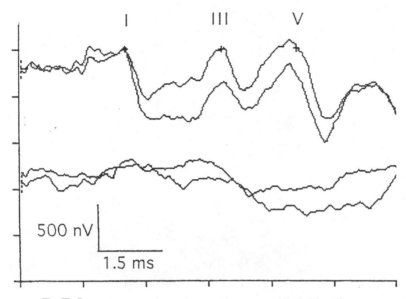

Figure 2-21 ABR recordings from a five-year-old child with one normal ear and one unresponsive ear.

When to Perform AABR Screening

AABR screening is generally performed as part of an institutional infant hearing screening protocol. It is less well suited than OAEs for screening children on an individual basis, for example, in a pediatrician's office, because valid assessment requires the child to be in a sleeping or restful state. Moreover, these devices are typically calibrated only for infants up to approximately six months of age.

When used in the newborn nursery, most programs obtain AABRs prior to discharge because of the difficulties encountered with follow-up and scheduling of return visits. As with OAE screening, there is no universal agreement regarding the best time to inform families of newborn hearing screening outcomes. While most programs inform parents at the time of hospital discharge, some choose to inform parents via written communication following discharge. Unfortunately, communication from hospital to home is often difficult, especially when there are linguistic barriers. Furthermore, parents may become upset if not informed immediately of any concerns regarding the results of hearing screening. See Parts II and III of this text for further discussion of communication with families.

Target Populations for AABR Screening

AABRs are well suited for infant screening. Specifically:

- Newborn infants in a well-baby nursery (i.e., universal infant hearing screening).
- High-risk infants in a special care nursery.
- High-risk infants not previously screened for hearing loss.

AABR screening is *not* recommended:

- For children with signs of acute otitis media, otorrhea, or other ear disease needing immediate medical attention.
- When the child is not sleeping or in a restful state.

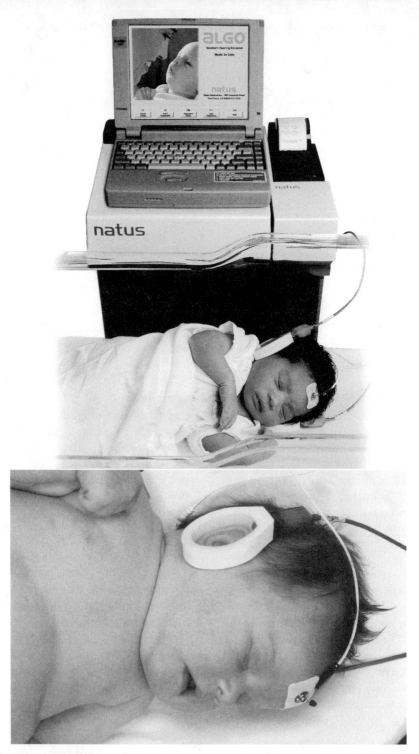

Figure 2-22 Infants undergoing automated ABR recording (top panel courtesy of Natus).

Personnel for AABR Screening

Professionals and support personnel from many disciplines have used AABRs successfully for screening. In the newborn nursery, AABR screening is often performed by a nurse. In other settings, support personnel conduct the screening. As with OAEs, it is strongly recommended that institutional screening programs be conducted under the general supervision of an audiologist. It is also important to ensure that personnel engaged in AABR screening are in full compliance with state licensure laws, scope of practice guidelines, and other regulatory requirements.

Test Environment for AABR Screening

Measurement of AABRs requires a relatively quiet environment and a site where equipment does not interfere with other activities. Many hospital nurseries have procedure rooms ideally suited for this activity and, in some, screening can be performed without moving the child out of the newborn nursery. Testing at maternal bedside has the same potential problems noted for OAE screening: fluctuating noise levels and other disturbances. Since it takes only a few minutes to complete AABR testing, the procedure is most efficiently performed in the nursery. Fortunately, portable lightweight battery-powered instruments allow considerable flexibility in where screening is performed, as long as noise levels are not excessive.

Screening Protocol for AABR

1. Attach the electrodes and transducers according to the manufacturer's specifications for the instrument used.
2. Record the screening results.
3. Arrange for referral/follow-up, as needed.

Referral and Follow-up

Children with possible hearing loss based on AABR should be referred to an audiologist. Some programs perform rescreening prior to referral. Careful consideration must be given to how and when parents are informed of the screening results (see Parts II and III of this text).

AABR Pitfalls and Practical Considerations

- Minimize room noise as much as possible.
- Exercise care when applying electrodes to avoid injury to the skin. Prepping the skin prior to electrode placement is usually unnecessary. A simple gauze wipe with soap and water is usually sufficient for an oily or hirsute infant.
- Conduct newborn screening early in the morning when there is less activity in the nursery.
- Infants who are bathed, fed, and sleepy tend to require the shortest test times.
- Swaddling infants in a nursery blanket allows them to remain in their preferred comfortable position.
- Be sure the infant meets the inclusion criteria for the device employed. For example, a gestational age of 34 weeks up to a chronological age of six months is typical. Also assumed is normal external ear anatomy, no use of CNS stimulant medications, an open crib, and a calm or sleeping infant.

- Be sure that sound transducers are attached exactly according to manufacturer's recommendations. In addition to delivering the stimulus, they attenuate ambient noise. Inappropriate placement will increase test time and referral rates.
- Transducers or electrodes designed for single use should not be reused.
- Electrode placement is critical. Be sure to attach electrodes exactly according to manufacturer's specifications.
- Automated ABR devices are designed for "hands-off" performance. Left alone, the screener will monitor impedance, ambient noise, and interference from muscle contraction. There is usually no need to intervene or disturb the infant unless prompted by the screening instrument to do so.
- Only complete tests should be considered valid.

SCREENING FOR OTITIS MEDIA

Tympanometry and Related Measures

Identification of otitis media is accomplished using *tympanometry* and related measures of tympanic membrane and middle ear mobility. They also provide information regarding middle ear pressure and equivalent volume. Taken together, the tests comprise a battery of middle ear screening procedures known as *acoustic immittance measures.*

Immittance measures assess middle ear function indirectly by examining how the ear responds to a "probe tone" presented in the sealed ear canal. The amount of acoustic energy "admitted" through the tympanic membrane and middle ear system is measured under various conditions described below. It should be noted that early instruments, instead of measuring the amount of acoustic energy admitted, measured the amount of energy reflected or "impeded" by the tympanic membrane and middle ear system. Thus, the term acoustic impedance was used to describe these early recordings. For a period of time, some instruments worked on the principle of acoustic impedance while others were based on acoustic admittance. As a result, the term "immittance" was coined to refer collectively to either measurement. While the general term acoustic immittance is still appropriate, modern instruments work on the principle of acoustic admittance. Thus, the term acoustic admittance or simply "admittance" will be used throughout the remainder of this chapter.

It is important to emphasize that acoustic admittance measures are *not* hearing tests. Rather, they are objective procedures used to provide information about the mechanical characteristics of the tympanic membrane and middle ear. The results obtained are then compared to those associated with normal middle ear function or various middle ear abnormalities. Because the prevalence of otitis media is low in older children and adults, middle ear screening is usually applied to young children through kindergarten age and older pediatric populations at increased risk.

As noted in Chapter 1, otitis media may be acute or it may occur in the form of otitis media with effusion (OME). Acute otitis media is usually characterized by pain, fever, and other overt symptoms that preclude the need for screening. It is the latter form, OME, which often exists without obvious symptoms (other than hearing loss) and, therefore, the condition likely to escape detection without systematic screening efforts. Because OME is a "silent" form of middle ear disease, the resulting hearing loss could be mistakenly attributed to attentional or developmental disorders.

Tympanometry

Tympanometry is an objective procedure used to evaluate the mechanical characteristics of the tympanic membrane and middle ear as pressure changes are created in the ear canal. The *tympanometer* emits a low frequency tone (typically 220 or 226 Hz) from a probe assembly placed in the ear canal (see Figures 2–23 and 2–24). Once the probe tip is sealed in the ear canal, the instrument creates a condition of either positive or negative pressure by pumping air in or out of the external ear canal. This allows the instrument to sample the mobility of the tympanic membrane and middle ear over a range of pressure conditions. Maximum mobility occurs when the air pressure created in the ear canal is equal to the air pressure in the middle ear space.

The instrument produces a graphic representation of these measurements known as a *tympanogram* (see Figure 2–25). When there is air in the middle ear space, the tympanogram will have a pressure peak that corresponds with the approximate air pressure in the middle ear space. Thus, the location of the peak provides an indirect estimate of middle ear pressure.

Tympanometric Peak Pressure, Equivalent Volume, and Static Admittance

Figure 2–26 shows a series of tympanograms and their interpretations. Referral criteria (ASHA, 1997) are provided in Table 2–6 and Table 2–7 for the measurements described below. The first tracing displayed, Figure 2–26A, shows a normal tympanogram with a peak at approximately zero. Note that air pressure, on the horizontal axis, is reported in decaPascals (daPa). The peak value of "−5" in Figure 2–26A indicates that middle ear pressure is approximately equal to the ambient air conditions, that is, the pressure in the surrounding environment. A normal middle ear will show pressure values ranging from approximately +50 to −150 daPa. A child with poor eustachian tube function caused by a cold, allergies, or upper respiratory infection may have *negative pressure* in the middle ear space. Such a condition is likely to produce a tympanogram with a negative peak (i.e., less than −150 daPa), like the one shown in Figure 2–26B. When tympanometry is performed on an ear with fluid in the middle ear space, the likely result is a "flat" tympanogram; that is, one that indicates little or no change in mobility as air pressure is varied in the ear canal (Figure 2–26C). When there is both air and fluid in the middle ear, or if an ear has reduced mobility caused by previous OME episodes, the resulting tympanogram may be "rounded." Such a tympanogram is shown in Figure 2–26D. Most tympanometers quantify the shape or sharpness of the peak by reporting it as a pressure interval (in daPa) that corresponds with a point equal to 50% of the admittance on either side of the peak, that is, half-way down the slope of the tympanogram on each side (see Figure 2–25). This measurement is labeled in Figure 2–26D as *tympanometric width*, although it should be noted that some instruments refer to this

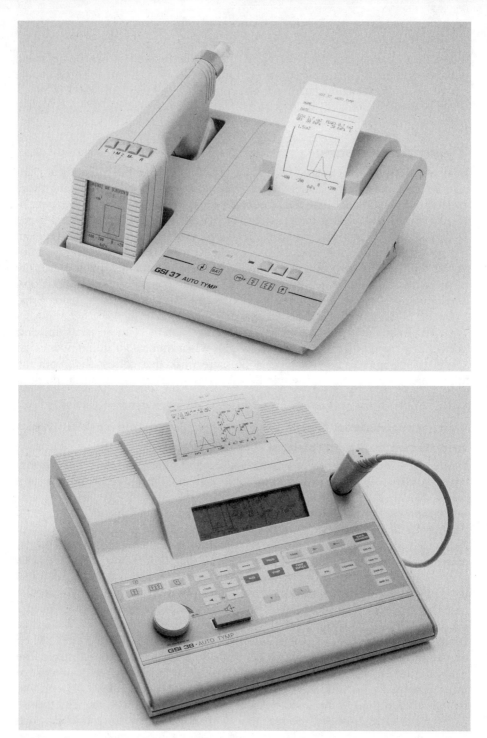

Figure 2-23 Portable tympanometers designed for middle ear screening: a cordless handheld device (A) and a combination tympanometer and acoustic reflex screener (B). (Courtesy of Grason-Stadler)

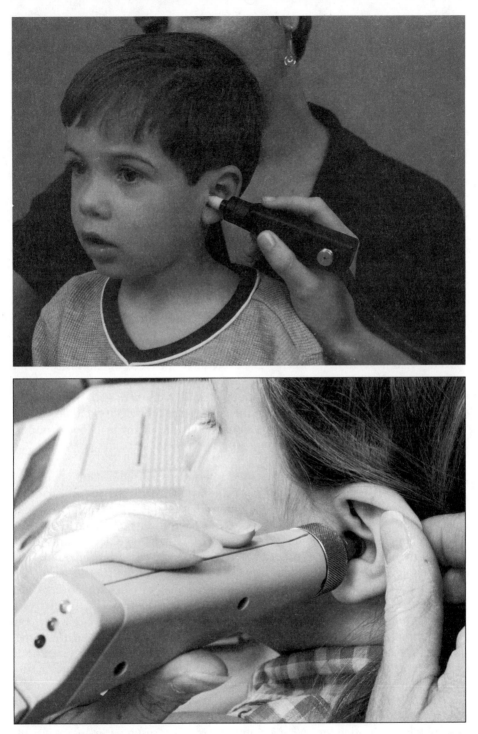

Figure 2-24 Placement of probe assembly for tympanometry. Younger children are often more at ease if seated in the lap of a parent or caretaker (A). Problems obtaining an airtight seal can often be solved by gently pulling the pinna up and back (B).

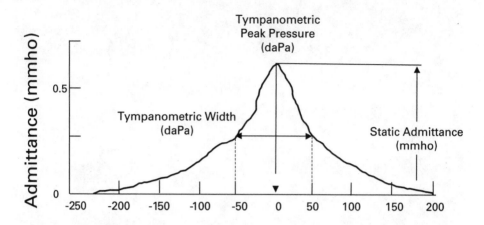

Figure 2-25 A normal tympanogram showing units of measurement according to ANSI standard S3.39–1987.

measurement as "gradient." Wide tympanograms are often difficult to interpret. Several studies have shown that broadly peaked, abnormally wide tympanograms, such as the one depicted in Figure 2–26D can occur when middle ear effusion is present. But wide tympanograms can also occur in the *absence* of middle ear effusion when the subject has a history of middle ear disease. Thus, when selecting pass-fail criteria it is important to choose "norms" based on populations with characteristics similar to those of the population targeted for screening.

The tympanometer can also be used to estimate the "equivalent volume" of the ear canal based on measurements of the probe tone in the sealed ear canal. When performed on a normal ear, the equivalent volume will be consistent with the amount of air space between the probe tip and the tympanic membrane. In contrast, an ear with a perforation of the tympanic membrane or a patent (open) tympanostomy tube would produce a tympanogram indicating an equivalent volume (air space) that includes both the ear canal *and* the middle ear space. Since the pressure changes created in the ear canal would have no effect on tympanic membrane mobility, the resulting tympanogram would be flat (see Figure 2–26E). Note that the tympanograms in Figures 2–26C and 2–26E are both flat, differing only with respect to the equivalent volume. That is, Figure 2–26C, with a normal volume, is suggestive of middle ear effusion while Figure 2–26E, with an abnormally large volume, suggests a perforation or a patent tympanostomy tube. Thus, estimates of ear canal volume are useful in screening for a perforation of the tympanic membrane. Equivalent volume estimates are also useful when checking the patency of a tympanostomy tube. In either case, the space in the middle ear is added to the space in the ear canal, resulting in an abnormally large equivalent volume. Still a third variant of the flat tympanogram would be one showing an abnormally *small* ear canal volume. Such a tympanogram might occur when the probe tip is against the ear canal wall or occluded by cerumen. Many of the devices used for tympanometric screening display an error message when the equivalent volume measurement is abnormally reduced. Others

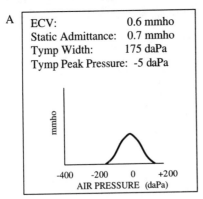

A

ECV:	0.6 mmho
Static Admittance:	0.7 mmho
Tymp Width:	175 daPa
Tymp Peak Pressure:	-5 daPa

Description
Equivalent Ear Canal Volume WNL
Middle Ear Mobility WNL
Middle Ear Pressure WNL

Interpretation
Normal Middle Ear Function

Follow-up
None

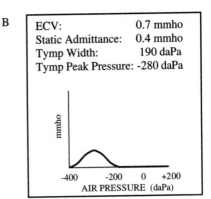

B

ECV:	0.7 mmho
Static Admittance:	0.4 mmho
Tymp Width:	190 daPa
Tymp Peak Pressure:	-280 daPa

Description
Equivalent Ear Canal Volume WNL
Slightly Reduced Mobility
Negative Middle Ear Pressure

Interpretation
Poor Eustachian Tube Function or
Normal Variability of Middle Ear
Pressure

Follow-up
None

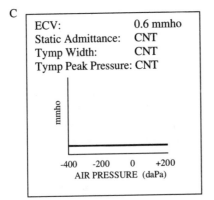

C

ECV:	0.6 mmho
Static Admittance:	CNT
Tymp Width:	CNT
Tymp Peak Pressure:	CNT

Description
Equivalent Ear Canal Volume WNL
Flat Tympanogram

Interpretation
Immobile TM/Middle Ear
Consistent with OME

Follow-up
Rescreen in 6-8 weeks (see text)

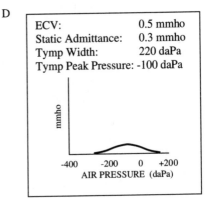

D

ECV:	0.5 mmho
Static Admittance:	0.3 mmho
Tymp Width:	220 daPa
Tymp Peak Pressure:	-100 daPa

Description
Equivalent Ear Canal Volume WNL
Wide Tympanogram
Low Mobility of TM/Middle Ear

Interpretation
Ambiguous: May be effusion

Follow-up
Rescreen in 6-8 weeks (see text)

Figure 2-26 A-D Tympanograms and related measures of acoustic admittance. ECV = equivalent ear canal volume; CNT = could not test; TM = tympanic membrane; WNL = within normal limits.

E

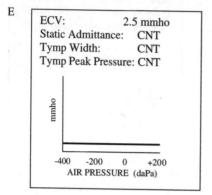

F

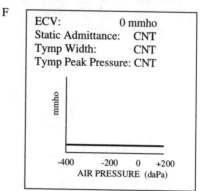

Description	Description
Abnormally Large Equivalent Volume	Abnormally Small Equivalent Volume
Flat tympanogram	Flat tympanogram
Interpretation	**Interpretation**
Possible TM Perforation or	Excessive Cerumen, Blocked Probe, or
Patent (open) Tympanostomy Tube	Probe Tip Against Canal Wall
Follow-up	**Follow-up**
Medical Referral (see text)	Inspect and Re-Position Probe or Refer
	for Ear Cleaning

Figure 2-26 E-F Tympanograms and related measures of acoustic admittance.

produce a flat tympanogram and report zero equivalent volume, as shown in Figure 2–26F. If the reduced volume is casued by inadequate probe placement, the device should be removed and re-inserted. If caused by excessive cerumen, the child must be referred for ear cleaning before a valid tympanogram can be obtained.

In summary, estimates of equivalent volume are essential because flat tympanograms may be the result of: 1) perforation of the tympanic membrane, a condition that would show an abnormally large equivalent volume estimate; 2) OME, which would result in a normal ear canal volume estimate; or 3) occlusion of the probe tip, which would show an abnormally small equivalent volume (or in some instruments a warning light or error message). There is one caution, however, that must be exercised in the interpretation of flat tympanograms: a normal equivalent volume does not rule out a perforation of the tympanic membrane. This is because the middle ear may contain effusion or

TABLE 2-6 Equivalent ear canal volume for children 1 to 7 years of age prior to and following placement of tympanostomy tubes.[1] (ASHA, 1997)

90% range for ears with and without tubes	Pretube equivalent volume	Post-tube equivalent volume
Fifth percentile–95th percentile	0.3–0.9 cm³	1.0–5.5 cm³

[1] *Shanks, Stelmachowicz, Beauchaine, and Schulte, 1992.*

TABLE 2-7 Referral criteria from ASHA (1997) for tympanometric width and peak static admittance (mmho = millimhos; daPa = decaPascals).

Infants[a]	One year to school age[b]
Static Admittance <0.2 mmho	Static Admittance <0.3 mmho[1]
or Tympanometric Width >235 daPa	or Tympanometric Width >200 daPa

[a]*Infants: Roush, Bryant, Mundy, Zeisel, & Roberts, 1995.*
[b]*Older children: Nozza, Bluestone, Kardatzke, & Bachman, 1992; 1994.*
[1]*For children >6 years of age, when using ±400 daPa for compensation of ear canal volume, peak static admittance <0.4 mmho is the recommended criterion.*

other space-occupying debris, even in the presence of a perforation. It may be assumed, however, that an ear with a flat tympanogram and an abnormally large equivalent volume is at risk for perforation. This finding is also consistent with a patent tympanostomy tube; however, children already receiving medical management for a middle ear problem are usually excluded from tympanometric screening (see recommended protocol, below).

The discussion of tympanometry to this point has been limited to admittance measures obtained in conjunction with air pressure variations in the ear canal. The tympanometer also provides information regarding middle ear admittance obtained from "static" or fixed measures of middle ear mobility. *Static admittance*, which is measured in *acoustic millimhos* (mmho), is calculated by measuring the height of the tympanometric peak and comparing it to one of its tail values (see Figure 2–25). Note that the tympanograms in Figures 2–25 and 2–26 are scaled on the vertical axis in millimhos (mmho). Infants and toddlers, especially those with histories of middle ear disease, usually demonstrate low peak static admittance even when middle ear effusion is not present. Since middle ear effusion reduces the mobility of the middle ear mechanism, tympanograms obtained from children with histories of recurrent OME are often characterized by low static admittance (Figure 2–26D). As explained earlier, an ear with OME is likely to produce a flat tympanogram because the middle ear is rendered immobile by the presence of effusion. Note that the tympanogram in Figure 2–26C, typical of that seen in OME, has markedly reduced static admittance.

The Acoustic Reflex

The *acoustic reflex*, also known as the stapedial (middle ear muscle) reflex, occurs when a high intensity sound causes contraction of the stapedius muscle, momentarily reducing the transmission of sound through the middle ear conductive mechanism and thereby lowering the sound levels reaching the inner ear. The acoustic reflex occurs in response to any loud sound and may serve to protect the inner ear and/or improve hearing in noisy situations. When the acoustic reflex is used clinically, it is elicited by a pure tone delivered via the tympanometer's probe assembly. Instruments designed for middle ear screening typically deliver an ipsilateral (same-ear) 1000 Hz pure tone through the probe assembly at levels ranging from 85 to 105 dB HL. The acoustic reflex is generally absent in an ear with middle ear dysfunction because the conductive hearing loss reduces the level of the acoustic stimulus reaching the inner ear and/or because the mechanical alterations caused by the middle ear disorder prevent it from being measured. Inclusion of the acoustic reflex has been shown by some studies to improve the identification of ears with otitis media, but this often occurs at the expense of lower specificity; that is, a higher number of false positive referrals.

The acoustic reflex has numerous applications when used clinically by the audiologist, but there is also a potential application in screening for middle ear effusion when it is necessary to interpret an ambiguous tympanogram. To explain, a flat tympanogram is generally expected when middle ear effusion is present and in such cases the acoustic reflex will be absent. But as noted earlier, middle ear effusion can be present even when the tympanogram has an identifiable peak, especially in cases of abnormally rounded or wide tympanograms. Since the acoustic reflex will most often be absent if middle ear fluid is present, the reflex can assist in differentiating wide tympanograms associated with effusion from those not associated with effusion. Unfortunately, mild middle ear abnormalities, such as negative middle ear pressure, may prevent detection of the acoustic reflex. Movement of the subject can also obscure reflex recording. As a result, several studies have shown an unacceptable over-referral rate when the acoustic reflex is included in a large-scale screening program. Thus, the acoustic reflex has limitations in an institutional screening program, but it remains potentially useful with a cooperative child in a well-controlled clinical environment, as a means of differentiating "borderline" tympanograms.

Automated Tympanometric Screening

Automated instruments for middle ear screening are available from many different manufacturers and most comply with ANSI standards. Figure 2–27 shows the output of two commercially available screening devices. Note that results are displayed differently. For example, some instruments use milliliters (ml) or cubic centimeters (cc) instead of mmho. For screening instruments, these three units of measure (ml, cc, mmho) can be considered equivalent. Both instruments in Figure 2–27 include each of the measurements described above.

Target Populations for Middle Ear Screening

The prevalence of OME is highest during the early months of life and decreases steadily throughout the preschool years. For typically developing children the prevalence of OME in children above the age of six years is very low. Consequently, most programs engaged in OME screening focus their efforts on older infants, toddlers, and preschool-age children, especially those with characteristics that place them at increased risk for OME

- Young children in group daycare.
- Children frequently exposed to cigarette smoke.
- Children with family histories of recurrent OME.
- Children with craniofacial anomalies associated with middle ear dysfunction such as Down syndrome or cleft palate.
- Children with histories of early onset acute otitis media (before 6 months of age).
- Racial groups known to have a high prevalence of OME, e.g., Eskimos and Native Americans.

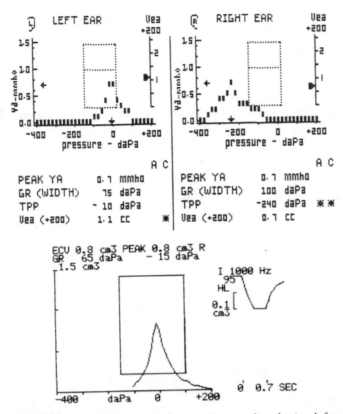

Figure 2-27   Tympanometric screening results obtained from two commercially available middle ear screeners. Differences in reporting of screening results are illustrated in these examples. In the upper figure, the left ear tympanogram is within normal limits for tympanometric peak pressure ("TPP"), equivalent volume ("Vea"), and tympanometric width ["GR (WIDTH)"]. The right ear demonstrates negative peak pressure (−240 daPa) but all other measures are within normal limits. The lower figure shows the output from another screener, this one providing acoustic reflex as well as tympanometric screening. Equivalent volume ("ECV") in the lower figure is reported in cubic centimeters (cm³), as is static admittance, which is labeled "PEAK." Tympanometric width, reported in daPa, is described as gradient ("GR").

Middle ear screening is *not* recommended:

- When there are signs or symptoms of acute otitis media or other ear disease.
- When otoscopic inspection reveals impacted cerumen or a foreign object.
- When excessive movement or lack of cooperation precludes valid assessment.
- For infants under 3 months of age.
- For children with tympanostomy tubes or those already being treated medically for middle ear disease.

Personnel for Tympanometric Screening

Tympanometric screening can be performed by a wide range of qualified health care providers; for example, nurses, pediatricians, speech-language pathologists, support personnel. Large-scale institutional screening programs should be conducted under the general supervision of an audiologist. State licensure laws, institutional policies, and guidelines for professional scope of practice should be reviewed to ensure that screening personnel are properly qualified and fully credentialed.

Test Environment for Tympanometric Screening

Tympanometric screening can be performed wherever there is sufficient space and lighting. A clean, uncluttered environment, free of unwanted distractions, is always preferable, but since a quiet environment is not a necessity, tympanometry can be carried out wherever it is most convenient. Portable, battery-operated devices, such as the one shown in Figure 2–28, allow considerable flexibility in the selection of a screening site.

Screening Protocol for Tympanometry

Every screening protocol must be carefully evaluated in the setting where it is used. The following protocol provides a useful starting point for most settings. When conditions permit inclusion of the acoustic reflex, the sensitivity of the middle ear screening protocol may be improved, but, as noted earlier, practitioners should consider the risk of over-referral when the acoustic reflex is included in large-scale institutional screening programs. Those responsible for the man-

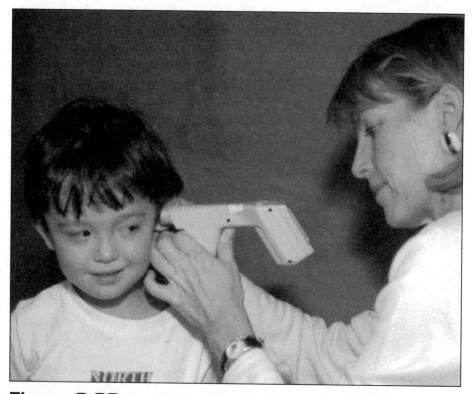

Figure 2-28 Portable, battery-operated devices, such as the one shown here, allow flexibility in the selection of a screening site.

agement of the program should systematically acquire data on screening outcomes to evaluate the suitability of a given screening protocol for the target population of interest. It must be emphasized that the overall success of a middle ear screening protocol will be enhanced considerably if the health care providers to whom referrals will be made (e.g., pediatricians and nurse practitioners) are actively involved in the design and evaluation of the program.

Tympanometry Procedures

1. Perform visual and otoscopic inspection of the external ear and ear canal. In the event of complete occlusion (impacted cerumen), foreign object, or signs of active ear disease (e.g., drainage from the ear canal), refer for medical management before proceeding. Referral is also indicated if there is evidence of disease, injury, or malformation of the outer ear.
2. Seat the child near the tympanometer. Explain what will occur: "I'm going to place this soft tip in your ear (show probe tip and probe assembly). You will hear some sounds, but all you need to do is hold still while the machine draws a picture with your ear. Be sure to hold still so we get a good picture."
3. Place the probe in the child's ear and obtain the measurements.
4. Record and interpret the results. Referral criteria (Tables 2–6 and 2–7) are as follows:

   Immediate medical referral when:

   • The equivalent volume estimate exceeds 1.0 mmho in the presence of a "flat" tympanogram (may indicate perforation of the tympanic membrane).

   Rescreening in 6–8 weeks when:

   • Static admittance is ≤0.2 mmho (includes all "flat" tympanograms) and/or
   • Tympanometric width ≥235 daPa for infants 6 mo to 1 yr or ≥200 for older children.

   At the time of rescreening, refer for medical review when:

   • Static admittance and/or tympanometric width are again abnormal.
5. Arrange for referral/follow-up, as needed.

Interpretation and Follow-Up

Children suspected of otitis media or other outer/middle ear disorders should be referred to their pediatrician or family practice physician. In some cases, when there is a history of chronic or recurrent middle ear disease, direct referral to an otolaryngologist may be warranted; however, many insurance policies and managed care providers require initial review and referral by a primary care physician.

Immediate medical referral is indicated for:

• Ear pain (*otalgia*);
• Discharge from the ear (*otorrhea*);
• Evidence of tympanic membrane perforation based on otoscopy and/or admittance measures; other evidence of ear disease.

Many children referred for medical review will not require immediate medical treatment. Most will be referred for suspected OME based on abnormal tympanometric findings. Although a referral of this nature is less urgent than a referral for one of the acute conditions described above, timely review is essential.

Physicians vary widely in their management of OME. Some will choose to follow the child for one or more return visits since the probability of spontaneous recovery is high. Others may choose a prophylactic course of antibiotics since the incidence of acute otitis media is higher when OME is already present. The Agency for Health Care Policy and Research (AHCPR) recommends referral to an otolaryngologist for consideration of tympanostomy tubes when OME persists for more than three months in the presence of bilateral hearing loss greater than 20 dB HL.

Regardless of whether referral is made for acute otitis media or OME, rescreening should be provided upon completion of medical treatment. It is not unusual for residual fluid to remain in the middle ear after an infection has been successfully treated with antibiotics. That is, while the acute symptoms may resolve, significant hearing loss may persist. A child should not be cleared until at least one normal follow-up evaluation has been observed. Additional information regarding referral, follow-up, and communication with families is provided in Part III of this text.

Tympanometry Pitfalls and Practical Considerations

- The ear canal should be inspected with an otoscope before placement of the probe assembly. Tympanometry should not be attempted when there is a foreign body in the ear canal.
- The probe tip should be carefully inspected for cerumen or other debris prior to each test. If the ports are occluded, consult the operation manual for proper cleaning.
- A valid tympanogram cannot be obtained on an ear canal occluded with cerumen; partial occlusion is usually not a problem.
- The child's movement and vocalizations should be minimized as much as possible since they can affect test results. A video player or other distraction device can be very helpful.
- "Flat" tympanograms require careful examination of equivalent volume estimates for accurate interpretation.
- The probe tip should provide a snug fit in the ear canal. Failure to acquire an adequate seal will increase test time and preclude some measurements.
- In general, it is best to repeat the tympanometric measures at least once to confirm consistency of test results.
- Tympanometric screening can be performed at any time; however, group screening is best performed in the fall of the year.
- In general, tympanometry should be used in conjunction with pure tone audiometry.

SUMMARY

Qualified personnel, using screening methods appropriately matched to the goals of a screening program, can successfully identify hearing loss and otitis media in children from infancy through school age. Identification of hearing loss in children at or below the developmental age of 5–6 months requires the use of physiologic test procedures: otoacoustic emissions and/or auditory brainstem responses. Thus, infant hearing screening, whether performed with a high-risk population in a neonatal intensive care unit or applied to all infants in a program of universal newborn hearing screening, requires use of one or both of these physiologic methods. A variety of screening personnel, working under the general supervision of an audiologist, can successfully employ these procedures.

For infants at a developmental level of approximately 6–30 months, behavioral hearing screening is possible; however, use of visual reinforcement audiometry requires expertise and a specialized testing environment typically found only in an audiology clinic. Consequently, this procedure is advocated for use by an audiologist or under the direct supervision of an audiologist. As a result, visual reinforcement audiometry for large-scale screening programs in this age group is unfeasible. Fortunately, otoacoustic emissions provide a physiologic alternative to behavioral screening for young children. This allows hearing screening to be performed during well-child visits in the pediatric office or in other settings where VRA is unfeasible or otherwise less desirable. Even so, when parents or caretakers have concerns about hearing in an infant or toddler, or when a child in this age group is being evaluated for special services, hearing assessment by an audiologist is warranted.

For children at a developmental level of 3–5 years, hearing screening of most children can be accomplished using behavioral pure tone "play" audiometry. This procedure is successfully employed in many settings by qualified nurses, speech-language pathologists, support personnel, and others. Again, otoacoustic emissions are a useful adjunct to behavioral screening, especially when evaluating children unwilling or unable to participate in behavioral procedures. It must be kept in mind, however, that physiologic tests are not "hearing tests" in the perceptual sense. They do, however, provide valuable information that is associated with normal or disordered hearing. Behavioral screening procedures (e.g., visual reinforcement audiometry or play audiometry) assess the auditory system at all levels, but they only provide information regarding hearing sensitivity.

Screening for otitis media is best accomplished using tympanometry and related measures. While these procedures are highly sensitive to middle ear dysfunction, they should not be viewed as diagnostic tools. Consequently, tympanometric screening results should be described as "consistent with middle ear effusion" or "suggestive of otitis media," when reported to parents or when referrals are made to health care providers. It should also be noted that measures of acoustic admittance are not useful as a method of detecting hearing loss. Rather, they should be used in conjunction with hearing screening measures when the goal is to identify otitis media as well as hearing loss. In the future, otoacoustic emissions will likely play a growing role in the identification of both hearing loss *and* middle ear dysfunction. Wide band reflectance is another technique that shows promise as a method of screening for middle ear effusion; however, further research and development are needed. Table 2–8 provides a summary of the procedures advocated in this chapter and their applications to hearing and middle ear screening in children. Part II of this text provides practical examples of how these procedures are applied in several

TABLE 2-8 Summary of methods used to screen for hearing loss and otitis media in children.

Screening method	Description	Purpose	Target populations	Comment
Otoacoustic Emissions (TEOAEs and DPOAEs)	Objective screening procedure based on physiologic assessment of cochlear function; recorded from a sensitive microphone in the ear canal.	Detection of hearing loss (also sensitive to middle ear effusion).	Newborn infants or older children when behavioral screening is unfeasible or less desirable.	Not sensitive to auditory neuropathy. May not detect mild sensory hearing loss.
Automated Auditory Brainstem Responses (AABRs)	Objective screening procedure based on physiologic assessment of auditory nerve and brainstem pathway; recorded from electrodes attached to the head.	Detection of hearing loss.	Newborn infants in a NICU or well-baby nursery.	Older children or those needing diagnostic ABR should be referred to an audiologist.
Visual Reinforcement Audiometry (VRA)	Behavioral screening procedure based on conditioned head-turn responses to frequency-specific auditory stimuli presented in a calibrated sound room.	Detection of hearing loss.	Infants/toddlers within a developmental age range of approximately 6–30 months.	Should be performed by, or under the direct supervision of, an audiologist (also see comment re: behavioral pure tone screening).
Behavioral Pure Tone Screening	Behavioral screening procedure based on "play" responses to frequency-specific auditory stimuli presented via earphones in a quiet listening environment.	Detection of hearing loss.	Toddlers and preschoolers within a developmental age range of approximately 3–5 years.	Will not detect hearing loss above or below screening frequencies; will not detect hearing loss below the screening level.
Acoustic Admittance (tympanometry)	Objective screening procedure based on TM/middle-ear response to a low frequency tone presented via a probe assembly sealed in the ear canal.	Detection of otitis media or perforation of the tympanic membrane.	Infants older than three months, including preschool and early elementary grade levels.	Not sensitive to hearing loss; should be used in conjunction with an appropriate hearing screening procedure.

model programs, in different settings, and with children in different age groups. Part III addresses the issues of referral, follow-up, and communication with families.

REFERENCES

Agency for Health Care Policy and Research. (1995). *Using clinical practice guidelines to evaluate quality of care* (Vol. 2, Methods, AHCPR Publication No. 95–0046). Washington, DC: Public Health Service, U.S. Department of Health and Human Services.

American Academy of Audiology. (1997). Report and Position Statement: Identification of hearing loss and middle ear dysfunction in preschool and school-age children. *Audiology Today, 9*(3), 18–23.

American National Standards Institute. (1987). *Specifications for instruments to measure aural acoustic impedance and admittance (aural acoustic immittance)* (ANSI S3.39–1987). New York: ANSI.

American National Standards Institute. (1991). *Criteria for permissible ambient noise during audiometric testing* (ANSI S3.1–1991). New York: ANSI.

American National Standards Institute. (1996). *Specification for audiometers* (ANSI S3.6–1996). New York: ANSI.

American Speech-Language-Hearing Association. (1990). Guidelines for screening for hearing impairment and middle ear disorders. *ASHA, 32*(Suppl. 2) 17–24.

American Speech-Language-Hearing Association. (1997). *Guidelines for audiologic screening.* Rockville, MD: ASHA.

Bluestone, C. D., Klein, J. O., & Kenna, M. A. (Eds.). 1990. *Pediatric otolaryngology* (3rd ed.). Philadelphia: Saunders.

Finitzo, T., Albright, K., & O'Neal, J. (1998). The newborn with hearing loss: Detection in the nursery. *Pediatrics, 102*, 1452–1460.

Friel-Patti, S., & Finitzo, T. (1990). Language learning in a prospective study of otitis media with effusion. *Journal of Speech Hearing Research, 33*, 188–194.

Glattke, T. J., Pafitis, I. A., Cummiskey, C., & Herer, G. R. (1995). Identification of hearing loss in children using measures of transient otoacoustic emission reproducibility. *American Journal of Audiology, 4*, 71–86.

Gravel, J. S., & Hood, L. J. (1999). Pediatric audiologic assessment. In F. E. Musiek & W. F. Rintelmann (Eds.), *Contemporary perspectives in hearing assessment* (pp. 305–326). Boston: Allyn & Bacon.

Gravel, J., Berg, A., Bradley, M., Cacace, A., Campbell, D., Dalzell, L., DeCristofaro, J., Greenberg, E., Gross, S., Orlando, M., Pinheiro, J., Regan, J., Spivak, L., Stevens, F., & Prieve, B. (2000). The New York State universal newborn hearing screening demonstration project: Effects of screening protocol on inpatient outcome measures. *Ear and Hearing, 21*, 131–140.

Hall, J. W. (2000). *Handbook of otoacoustic emissions.* San Diego: Singular Thomson Learning.

Henderson, F., & Roush, J. (1997). Identification and diagnosis of otitis media with effusion. Chapter 2, pp. 43–59. In J. Roberts, I. Wallace, & F. Henderson (Eds.), *Otitis media, language, and learning in young children.* Baltimore: Paul H. Brookes.

Herrmann, B., Thornton, A., & Joseph, J. (1995). Automated infant screening using the ABR: Development and evaluation. *American Journal of Audiology, 4*, 6–14.

Joint Committee on Infant Hearing. (2000). Joint committee on infant hearing 2000: Position statement. *Audiology Today,* August, Special Issue, 6–27.

Kenna, M. A. (1990). Embryology and developmental anatomy of the ear. In Bluestone, C. D., Klein, J. O., Kenna, M. A. (Eds.), *Pediatric otolaryngology* (3rd ed.). Philadelphia: Saunders.

Lonsbury-Martin, B. L., Whitehead, M. L., & Martin, G. K. (1991). Clinical applications of otoacoustic emissions. *Journal of Speech and Hearing Research, 34*(5), 964–981.

Margolis, R. H., & Heller, J. (1987). Screening tympanometry: Criteria for medical referral. *Audiology, 26*, 197–208.

Nozza, R. J. (1995). Critical issues in acoustic-immittance screening for middle-ear effusion. *Seminars in Hearing, 16*(1), 86–98.

Nozza, R. J., Bluestone, C. D., & Kardatzke, D. (1992). Sensitivity, specificity, and predictive values of immittance measures in the identification of middle-ear effusion. In F. H. Bess & J. W. Hall (Eds.), *Screening children for auditory function,* pp. 315–329. Nashville, TN: Bill Wilkerson Press.

Nozza, R. J., Bluestone, C. D., Kardatzke, D., & Bachman, R. (1994). Identification of middle ear effusion by aural acoustic admittance and otoscopy. *Ear and Hearing, 15(4)*, 310–323.

Roush, J., Bryant, K., Mundy, M., Zeisel, S., & Roberts, J. (1995). Developmental changes in static admittance and tympanometric width in infants and toddlers. *Journal of the American Academy of Audiology, 6(4)*: 334–338.

Shanks, J. E., Stelmachowicz, P. G., Beauchaine, K. L., & Schulte, L. (1992). Equivalent ear canal volumes in children pre- and post-tympanostomy tube insertion. *Journal of Speech and Hearing Research, 35(4)*, 936–941.

Stool, S. E., Berg, A. O., Berman, S., Carney, C. J., Cooley, J. R., Culpepper, L., Eavey, R. D., Feagans, L. V. Finitzo, T., & Friedman, E. (1994). *Managing otitis media with effusion in young children. Quick reference guide for clinicians* (AHCPR Publication No. 94–0623). Rockville, MD: Agency for Health Care Policy and Research, Public Health Service, U.S. Department of Health and Human Services.

Wiley, T. L., & Smith, P. S. (1995). Acoustic-immittance measures and middle-ear screening. *Seminars in Hearing, 16(1)*, 60–80.

Developmental Milestones for Speech, Language, and Communication

Elizabeth R. Crais, Ph.D.

INTRODUCTION

As the African proverb denotes, "It takes a village to raise a child," so like that proverb is the identification of young children who are at risk for or have communication or broad-based developmental deficits. All who come in contact with children have the opportunity and responsibility to be a part of that "village" to help in the identification process. Because of the role audiologists and other health care providers play in monitoring children's middle ear and hearing status, these professionals may be the first to suspect a developmental disability. Conversely, when a child is suspected of having a communication deficit, early concerns about hearing status may prompt interactions with audiologists and related health care professionals. Indeed, for children suspected (and later diagnosed) with certain types of disabilities (e.g., language deficits, pervasive developmental disorder, autism spectrum disorder), hearing loss is often one of the first risk factors investigated when trying to identify the cause for the deficit. So that all professionals who encounter children may be part of the "village," it is helpful to be familiar with background information and behaviors that may be indicators of communication and related deficits. Moreover, once a child has been identified as having communication difficulties, information about the developmental course of communication skills can be helpful when providing services to the child. This chapter presents some of the milestones and "red flags" that may help professionals and family members: 1) decide whether to refer a child for initial or further evaluation, 2) identify the key behaviors important for a child's communication and social development, and 3) to provide input for intervention planning.

ISSUES IN IDENTIFYING COMMUNICATION DEFICITS

Communication is the process of exchanging information, ideas, and/or feelings with others and is typically considered a social act. There are various forms of communication (e.g., verbal, such as sounds and words, and nonverbal, including gestures, body and facial movements). Many species communicate (e.g., bees, dogs, humans); however, few species have a mutually shared symbol system, which is required for communication to be considered *language*. Language can be transmitted in a variety of ways, such as speaking, writing, using sign language, or using picture symbols to represent meaning. Communication is present at birth (or before) and children communicate long before they learn to understand or speak the language that surrounds them. Within this chapter, the terms communication skills and communication deficits will be used predominantly to keep the focus off *language* skills, and to highlight the many additional ways children can communicate.

Communication deficits may occur alone or may be secondary to other types of disabilities, such as mental retardation, autism, or cerebral palsy. Much evidence exists to indicate that early communication delays or disorders may impact a child's social, cognitive, emotional, spoken and written language, reading, and later academic development. Given that 12% of all school-age children receive special education services, whereas only 4.4% of preschoolers and 1.4% of infants and toddlers receive early intervention services, the *early* identification of these children is critical (U.S. Department of Education, 1996).

Two approaches will be used within this chapter to highlight background information and behaviors necessary for identifying delays in a child's communication and related skill areas. The first uses the "typical" age when children acquire a particular *language comprehension* or *production* skill. The second examines multiple skill areas related to *communication* and identifies *upper limits* at which all children should have acquired a particular skill. Both methods can be useful and viewed as complementary types of information.

"Typical" Milestones Approach

The first approach is a more traditional way to look at development and uses milestones that "most" children should achieve to indicate what is "expected" of a particular child's development at each level. This approach is represented in Table 3–1, using key language comprehension and production milestones and the comparable age at which each skill is "typically" acquired by young children.

One of the major difficulties in identifying young children with communication deficits, however, has been the primary focus on specific language *production* markers, such as when the child begins to use words, the number of words in the production vocabulary, and the combination of words into sentences. Although these milestones are useful indicators for some children, for others they are less than definitive. For example, although many children use their first word around 12 months of age, first word use is quite variable, ranging from 8 to 20 months of age. The size of children's production vocabularies also varies considerably; with some typically developing 18-month-olds having no words, whereas others have over 500 words. Putting words together may also occur anywhere between 18 and 30 months in some children. Therefore, the extreme variability in what "typically developing" children do is problematic, and when children do not meet one or more of these key production milestones, the question is always, "Are they late bloomers or is there a real deficit?" Adding comprehension information does increase the likelihood of being able to recognize which children are more likely to be truly delayed, versus those who may be "late talkers." Indeed, there is a good bit of evidence that children who have deficits in both production and comprehension are more likely to display

TABLE 3-1 Children's milestones of communication development.

Age	Hearing/Understanding	Expressing
Birth to 3 months	• Can be quieted by a familiar, friendly voice • Startles, cries, or wakes when there is a loud sound	• Produces small, throaty noises
3 to 6 months	• Enjoys rattles and other sound-making toys • Responds to pleasant tones by cooing • Stops playing and appears to listen to sounds or speech	• Laughs out loud • Cries differently for pain, hunger, and discomfort • Coos—produces an assortment of oohs, ahs, and other vowel sounds
6 to 9 months	• Responds to soft levels of speech and other sounds • Temporarily stops action in response to "no" • Turns head directly toward voices and interesting sounds • Begins to understand routine words when used with a hand gesture (e.g., bye-bye or up)	• Babbles—repeats consonant-vowels combinations such as ba-ba-ba • Makes raspberry sound • Makes sounds with rising and falling pitches
9 to 12 months	• Follows simple directions presented with gestures (e.g., give it to me, come here) • Responds to his or her own name, even when spoken quietly • Will turn and find sound in any direction	• Vocalizes to get attention • Imitates sounds • Produces a variety of speech sounds (e.g., m, b, d) in several pitches
12 to 18 months	• Knows the names of familiar objects, persons, and pets • Follows routine directions presented without gestural or visual cues (e.g., come here, clap hands) • Identifies sounds coming from another room or outside • Enjoys music and may try to dance	• Uses 2 to 3 words spontaneously • Imitates simple words • Uses jargon speech (babbling that sounds like real speech) to communicate • Points to request or draw attention to objects, people, and events
18 to 24 months	• Points to two or more body parts • Identifies five or more pictures of common objects when named	• Uses vocabulary of 20+ words • Uses jargon speech with intelligible words • Says "no" or "no-no" in response to questions or commands
24 to 30 months	• Responds to two-part command (e.g., get the shoe and bring it to me) • Listens to simple stories • Understands possessive terms (my, mine, yours)	• Puts together two or more words to make simple sentences • Uses vocabulary of 50+ words • 50% of speech can be understood by unfamiliar listeners

Table 3–1 (*continued* on following page)

TABLE 3-1 (*continued* from previous page).

30 to 36 months	
• Answers to "what" and "who" questions • Identifies objects and pictures by use (e.g., show me what you sit on) • Easily follows simple conversation • Understands basic concepts (e.g., big, little, in, on)	• Consistently uses 2- to-3 word sentences • Asks "what" and "where" questions • Uses some plural (e.g., cars) and verb markers (e.g., running) • 50–75% of speech can be understood by unfamiliar listeners

Reprinted by permission. Bill Wilkerson Center Press, Nashville, TN.

continuing delays than children with "production only" deficits. However, there is also evidence that some children with early "delays" may test in the "typical" range at early school age.

An additional issue in identification is the limited scope of development actually covered by looking primarily at comprehension and production skills. As indicated previously, there is much more to communication skills than just the *language* components and, although some aspects of broader communication and related skills are addressed by milestone charts such as Table 3–1, other areas such as cognition, social interaction, play, and sound development are examined in a limited way.

Red Flags Approach Across Multiple Developmental Areas

An additional way to look at development is to examine a variety of developmental areas that may be at risk and to use an aggregate view of them to help determine the need for referral or the need to make accommodations in providing intervention services. Although a delay in one area does not in itself indicate a deficit, concerns in multiple areas provide professionals and family members with more certainty that further assessment is warranted and/or that more global interventions are needed. Moreover, taking an approach that attempts to indicate the uppermost limit at which *all* children should have acquired key skills can provide additional guideposts or "red flags" for helping in the decision making process. The following sections provide information across key developmental areas related to communication, along with potential "red flags" that may signal a need for referral.

SOCIAL INTERACTION

Increasing evidence indicates that the frequency and quality of young children's early social interactions are predictive of their later communicative development. Observing and asking about a young child's social skills can provide a wealth of information to professionals about both the child's current skills and his developmental potential. Early in life, infants show a readiness for social interaction through a variety of means. They may quiet when seeing a face or hearing a sound, they may look attentively at the source (e.g., lights, sounds, faces), and later they may become excited by seeing or hearing familiar faces or voices.

Clearly, they also may show displeasure at strangers or new environments. By 2–3 months, infants should be easily engaged by a familiar adult and should be smiling readily in response to caregivers. Children who do not demonstrate a social smile to a familiar adult by the age of 3 months are at risk for social/communication delays (see Table 3–2). By 4–8 months, infants should be attentive to familiar games or routines, and may be making gooing and cooing sounds to caregivers or others who talk to them. By 8 months, infants should be vocalizing back to adults (e.g., child vocalizes, adult vocalizes, child vocalizes again), but are not yet readily imitating adults. As children emerge into intentional communication (discussed in the next section) between 8 and 12 months, they should begin to show and give objects to others. Young children often delight in holding up or extending objects (particularly new or novel ones) to familiar adults. In essence the child is sharing the pleasure or curiosity of the object with the adult, and in this way brings the adult into the child's immediate realm of interest. The ability of the child to share attention with others to objects or events (e.g., jointly looking at object, book, or activity) typically emerges around 9 months; however, it may not be consistently displayed in some children until 15 months of age. By 15 months, children typically engage in pointing to objects of interest either to request the object or to comment nonverbally about it. If a child is not showing or giving objects to familiar adults by 12 months of age, or is not sharing joint attention or pointing by 15 months, there may be cause for concern. Inattentiveness to people, lack of eye contact, or lack of shared mutual gaze with familiar adults should all be signals of a child's risk for communication difficulties. Indeed, there is a high correlation between the amount of time spent in joint engagement with the caregiver and the child's later vocabulary skills (Carpenter, Nagell, & Tomasello, 1998).

For older infants and toddlers, interest in social interaction may be indicated by sustained eye contact, tolerance of being close to or engaged by a stranger, giving or showing or receiving objects, and/or vocalizations or verbalizations directed toward a family member or professional. For older children, social interaction may take many forms and caregivers should be able to describe the ways that their young child plays and interacts with them and others. Once children are ambulatory, games of chase or "I'm going to get you" are

TABLE 3-2 Red flags for social development.	
Be concerned if the child is *not*:	**By:**
Responding to familiar adults with a social smile	3 months
"Talking" back by vocalizing to familiar adults who talk to the child	8 months
Attentive to social games played by familiar adults (e.g., peek-a-boo)	8 months
Participating in social games (e.g., puts up hands for "patty-cake")	12 months
Showing and/or giving objects to familiar adults	15 months
Pointing to objects to indicate interest in them	18 months
Seeking adult interaction to play with toys/look at books	18 months
Pointing either spontaneously or by request to pictures in books	24 months

General social concerns: inattentiveness to people, lack of eye contact or shared mutual gaze with familiar adults by 12 months; preferring to play alone at 18 months or older; or when social play is limited to "chase" or "tickle" games at 24 months.

common. If parents report that chase or tickle games are among the few or only types of interactions their young children take part in, concerns about the child's social skills should be raised. Children 18–24 months love objects that they can manipulate (e.g., open, put in, take out, stack) and they should be readily seeking adult attention and help to play with these types of toys. Generally, young children up to three years of age prefer to play with adults and when parents relate that their child prefers to play alone, especially for long periods of time, red flags may be raised about the child's social and communicative development. By 24 months, most children should be able to look briefly at picture books with caregivers and point (either spontaneously or by request) to objects represented in the books. If parents report that their two-year-old child does not like looking at picture books alone or with them, be sure to ask the kind of books available to the child. For young children with expressive communication delays, parents may assume higher level skills because of the child's comprehension skills, and may be using books that may are too advanced for the child's production skills. A lack of interest in books by 24 months or preferring to look at them alone, may be additional indicators of risk. By asking the type of books children like, professionals can also gain perspective on the child's cognitive and communication skills. Board books and single picture per page books are often favored by young children 6–15 months. Fifteen-to-18-month-olds enjoy looking at simple action books (e.g., babies doing different things) and 24-month-olds can typically be engaged in very short action sequences (e.g., a child getting ready for bed). Three- and four-year olds should be able to attend to longer stories with characters participating in several events (e.g., child goes to preschool). By the age of five, children should not only be able to listen attentively to short stories, but should also be able to relate some of the events of the story to caregivers.

It is not unusual for young children to be hesitant around strangers and in new settings. Thus, professionals often need the report of caregivers or teachers to gain a picture of the child's *typical* interaction style in familiar surroundings. Asking caregivers to demonstrate the child's favorite social games (e.g., peek-a-boo, patty-cake), play with the child using toys, or perform book-reading activities may provide a window into the child's level of engagement with a familiar adult. Caregivers can also be an excellent resource for knowing what adult interaction style their child likes and may respond to best. If professionals suspect social interaction deficits, it is extremely important to observe the child in familiar settings and/or gather information from familiar adults about how the child interacts on a routine basis. Hesitancy in interacting with strangers is a normal developmental process and should not be assumed to be indicative of a deficit; however, as indicated by much of the literature, delays in social interaction often accompany (and may complicate the identification of) communication deficits.

INTENTIONALITY

Infants' early behaviors are not thought to be intentional, although they communicate states such as hunger, pain, or pleasure. It is through the caregivers' consistent responses to these behaviors that the child learns to associate certain behaviors with certain intents (e.g., crying results in being picked up). Typically between 6 and 12 months of age, children progress from using unintentional communicative behaviors to intentional behaviors that serve to directly affect another's behavior. Varied means of communication are available to the child and include vocalizations, eye gaze, body or facial gestures, word approximations, and words. Children in this early intentional stage communicate primarily to: 1) regulate someone else's behavior by making a request (e.g., reaching to be picked up) or protesting (e.g., pushing away undesired object); 2) achieve and maintain social interaction by using greetings, playing social games, such as peek-a-boo or patty-cake, gesturing, and showing off; and 3) draw attention to an object, event, or action (Wetherby & Prizant, 1993). These basic reasons for communicating predominate throughout the first two years of life, even as children gain more sophisticated ways to communicate (e.g., early gestures and vocalizations give way to the later use of words). Later developing intentions include requesting permission, acknowledging something said or done (e.g., nodding or saying "yes"), clarifying (e.g., pointing at an object while saying the word), and requesting information (usually through asking questions), and typically do not emerge until the one-word (12–20 months) or multiword (24+ months) stage (Wetherby & Prizant, 1993).

Twelve-month-olds typically communicate intentionally about one time per minute, using primarily gestures and vocalizations, 18-month-olds about two times per minute with a combination of gestures, vocalizations, and words or word approximations, and 24-month-olds about five times per minute using primarily words or word combinations (Wetherby, Cain, Yonclas, & Walker, 1988).

The first task for professionals and caregivers is to determine whether the child has reached an intentional stage of communication. Asking caregivers how and for what reasons a child communicates, and observing how the child gets his or her needs met can usually provide a basis for determining intentionality. Because determining intentionality is difficult with some children in the early stages, Wetherby and Prizant's (1993) criteria for judging intentionality may be helpful. For example, does the child: 1) alternate eye gaze between the listener and the goal; 2) persist in signaling (e.g., continue to fuss) or change the signal until the goal is accomplished (e.g., cry and then move arms and legs); 3) use a conventional signal (e.g., waving bye) or ritualized form (e.g., laying down on the floor to request diaper changing); 4) pause for a response from the listener; 5) stop signaling and/or display satisfaction when the goal is met, and 6) display dissatisfaction when the goal is not met? Red flags (see Table 3–3) should be raised for children who are 10 months of age or older who do not demonstrate

---

TABLE 3-3   Red flags for intentionality.

Be concerned if the child is *not:*	By:
Showing any type of intentional behavior (e.g., requesting, protesting)	10 months
Communicating for a variety of reasons (e.g., protesting, requesting, seeking social interaction, commenting)	18 months
Using a variety of means (e.g., gesturing, vocalizing, using eye gaze)	18 months

General intentionality concerns: children who primarily regulate others' behavior (e.g., putting someone's hand on toy to operate it, leading adult to door to open it), but do not display more social forms of communicating (e.g., giving book to another to read, pointing to objects of interest, drawing attention to self for social reasons).

any communicative intentions (especially protesting, which appears fairly early). In addition, children 12 to 18 months should be communicating for a variety of reasons (e.g., protesting, requesting, seeking social interaction, commenting) using a variety of means (e.g., gesturing, vocalizing, using eye gaze, and perhaps word approximations or words). Those 18–24-month-olds who display a low rate of communicating, limited reasons, and/or limited ways to communicate should be considered at risk. For certain groups of children (e.g., those with autism spectrum disorders), deficits in social interaction and intentionality are particularly strong characteristics of the disorder, and therefore may be early indicators of later diagnoses. Further, although these children may communicate frequently to regulate someone's behavior (e.g., pulling adult's hand or fussing to get the door open), they typically do not communicate for more social reasons (e.g., showing off, pointing to objects, bringing books for adults to look at with them). In addition, they often display a limited range of ways to communicate (e.g., little or no use of intentional vocalizations, gestures, eye contact, or words). Care should be taken not to assume a "diagnosis" based on intentionality alone; however, the information gained from looking at intentional development can be contributory in decision making.

PLAY SKILLS

For most children, play and communication skills are highly correlated during some stages of development, and both reflect common underlying cognitive processes. Therefore, by obtaining information about a child's play skills, professionals can make some assumptions about the child's communication and cognitive skills. Children in the first four months of life play by looking at, holding, and mouthing objects. By 4–8 months, as fine motor skills increase, play includes mouthing, banging, shaking, and manipulating objects (see Table 3–4). By 8–12 months, infants begin to manipulate objects more readily, throwing and dropping them, giving and showing them to adults, and begin to be participants in social games (e.g., patty-cake). At the 12–18 month level, toddlers typically push, pull, turn on, put in, and take out objects. They are beginning to stack objects and figure out the relationships between play objects. Between 18 and 24 months, toddlers are playing easily with a variety of toys (e.g., blocks, cars, dolls, sandbox toys, stuffed animals) and should be clearly showing their knowledge of how to use these toys functionally. By 24 to 36 months, more elaborate actions with objects should be displayed, such as figuring out how to open containers with screw lids, fitting simple shapes into their associated holes, and using pretend play.

Single pretend schemes (e.g., child eats from a play spoon) typically emerge between 12 and 20 months, along with first words. A child who is spontaneously demonstrating single pretend schemes may be showing a cognitive readiness for word approximations or words (depending on the other skills the child has available). Children who are 20–24 months old and are not exhibiting any pretend play behaviors may be at risk for communication deficits. Further, as children begin to combine words (20 to 24 months), single pretend schemes are typically joined together (e.g., child stirs pretend food and then feeds self). A child who is combining play behaviors but not words may be showing symbolic

TABLE 3-4 Red flags for play skills.	
Be concerned if the child is *not*:	**By:**
Mouthing, banging, shaking, and/or manipulating objects	8 months
Throwing, dropping toys, especially for others to get	12 months
Participating in social games (e.g., looks for Mom during "peek-a-boo")	12 months
Giving or showing toys to adults	15 months
Pushing, pulling, turning on, putting in, and taking out objects	18 months
Showing knowledge of how to use toys functionally (e.g., push toy car)	18 months
Stacking cups or rings on a ring stacker (not necessarily correctly)	24 months
Performing some pretend play behaviors (e.g., drinking from empty cup)	24 months
Combining play acts (e.g., rocks baby and puts down for nap)	30 months
Playing with familiar children some of the time when in close proximity	36 months
Taking turns in constructive or pretend play with familiar children	48 months

General play concerns: children who primarily perform play behaviors representative of younger children; have limited play behaviors (e.g., play with only one type of toy, play very briefly with toys); seem averse to playing with others (including caregivers); play alone for longer periods of time than would be expected at their developmental age; have stereotypic play behaviors (e.g., repeatedly opening and closing drawers, lining up their toys and becoming upset if others change the order); or display unusual play behaviors (e.g., rub plastic stacking rings over their hands or face, lick and smell toys).

readiness for word combinations. By 28 months, most children are producing longer sentences, sequencing their play actions, and play acting familiar scenarios. Three-year-olds are developing their ability to play actively with others, although for short periods of time, and are improving their ability to take turns. Four- and five-year-olds should be engaging in cooperative and pretend play by building together, enacting pretend scenarios, and taking turns readily.

Children are at risk for communication and other developmental deficits when they: primarily display play behaviors representative of younger children; have limited play behaviors (e.g., play with only one type of toy, play very briefly with toys); seem averse to playing with others (including caregivers); play alone for longer periods of time than would be expected at their developmental age (e.g., one hour for a 24-month-old); have stereotypic play behaviors (e.g., continuously spinning the wheels of a car, rigidly lining up their toys); or display unusual play behaviors (e.g., rub toys across their face or hands, lick and smell toys). Observation and caregiver report of a child's play behaviors can provide a baseline from which to make assumptions about the child's overall developmental level and, more specifically, about the child's potential for the development or refinement of associated communication skills.

LANGUAGE COMPREHENSION

For most children, comprehension skills exceed production skills. Most children are referred for evaluation because of their production deficits, yet a subset of these children will have deficits in comprehension as well. As noted, deficits in both areas place a child at greater risk than a child with production deficits only. In order to detect comprehension deficits in young children, both the child's non-linguistic response strategies (i.e., those based on information other than words) and later linguistic comprehension strategies (i.e., those based primarily on words) need to be addressed. In identifying the types of strategies that infants and toddlers use in comprehending their environment, Chapman's early work (1978) provides an excellent overview. Non-linguistic response strategies are what children use to comprehend events before they are able to use linguistic strategies. Early non-linguistic strategies used between 8 to 12 months include looking at objects looked at by others, acting on objects that are noticed, and imitating ongoing actions (see Table 3–5). Children continue to use non-linguistic strategies in the 12–18 month stage, such as doing what is usually done in a situation (e.g., child puts on coat when everyone else does); and in the 18–24 month stage, such as putting objects in containers or on surfaces (e.g., child puts block in box before examiner says, "Put the block in the box").

Using linguistic strategies depends on understanding some element of the linguistic message (e.g., child picks up a toy mentioned). Strategies used in the 12 to 18 month stage include attending to an object mentioned, and giving evidence of notice (e.g., child looks up when his/her name is called). In addition to those mentioned, linguistic strategies used from 18 to 24 months include locating an object mentioned, and acting on objects in the way mentioned (e.g., combing hair with comb). From 24–36 months, children use probable location (e.g., the child can recognize "Put the apple in the trash can," but not "Put the apple in your shoe.") or probable event strategies ("The mommy fed the baby," but not "The baby fed the mommy"). Children at this stage may also use a strategy to supply missing information; for example, if asked a question of any type, they may respond with their name.

To help in the determination of whether a referral is necessary for a young child, professionals should ask caregivers about the kinds of words and phrases their child will respond to and follow. Examples include: does the child respond to his/her own name or those of others? does the child look at an object named? and for older toddlers, can the child point to or go get an object named? and will the child comply with simple requests? (e.g., come here, give me the ball). By the age of one, most children should be responding by looking when their

TABLE 3-5 Red flags for comprehension skills.

Be concerned if the child is *not*:	By:
Looking at objects looked at by others	12 months
Acting on objects that are noticed	12 months
Imitating ongoing actions	12 months
Responding to own name	15 months
Attending to an object mentioned	15 months
Doing what is usually done in a situation (e.g., child puts on coat when others do)	18 months
Using conventional behaviors (e.g., combing hair with comb)	18 months
Acting on objects as the agent (e.g., child brushes own teeth when asked to "Brush the baby's teeth")	24 months
Responding to many object names	24 months
Retrieving a familiar object out of sight	24 months

name is called. By age two, children should be able to respond to many object names, two-step commands, and requests to retrieve a familiar object out of sight. Children's listening and comprehension skills can also be identified by asking parents about the type of books their children enjoy, and by gaining information on what types of questions and commands the child will follow during bookreading interactions. Development typically begins with "what" (What's that?), "where" (Where's the dog?) and "what doing" (What is she doing?) questions. For older children, questions about their ability to follow conversations, interact with peers and less familiar adults, and understand a variety of more complex questions asked of them (e.g., why, what if, when, how) may help shed light on any concerns about comprehension skills.

Because of the use by young children of non-linguistic response strategies and early linguistic strategies, comprehension problems are often difficult for caregivers and teachers to detect. Therefore, any mention by the caregiver or teacher of the possibility that a child may have a comprehension deficit should be pursued with observation and testing. When parents and/or teachers report "behavior problems" with a child, comprehension difficulties and hearing loss should always be a dual focus of attention. Similarly, as noted previously, when parents report that their child does not like looking at books or being read to, comprehension skills should be investigated.

SOUND PRODUCTION

When trying to make decisions about a child's overall communication level and whether a referral is necessary, looking at the child's sound-making capacities is important. As suggested by many, phonological development is often a better predictor of developmental level than is chronological age. Typically developing infants produce reflexive sounds for the first few months, move on to comfort or cooing sounds between 2 to 4 months, begin to produce longer series of syllables and prolonged vowels and consonants with much vocal play between 4 to 6 months, produce reduplicated babbling (e.g., bababa) between 7 to 9 months, and use more varied and complex babbling (e.g., badaba) and their first words somewhere after 10 months (Smith, Goffman, & Stark, 1995). In addition to the sound production items listed in Table 3–1, several key milestones have emerged in recent years (see Table 3–6). For example, the onset of true babbling (e.g., repeated sounds and syllables such as bababa, nunu) by 11 months of age is a key developmental marker and those children who do not babble by 11 months should be considered at risk, particularly for hearing loss (Eilers & Oller, 1994).

For young children, it is important to identify the child's level of sound-making development (e.g., type of vocalizations, word approximations, words), their breadth of sound-making capabilities at any one level, and their imitative ability. For example, a child may be producing word approximations, but with a very limited repertoire of syllable shapes or consonants and vowels (e.g., ba/ball, ba/bottle, ba/baby) and may be very hesitant to imitate other people. This child's overall prognosis may be poorer than that of a child who may not yet be producing word approximations, but who already uses jargon speech with a large range of consonants and vowels, produces varied types of syllables, and readily imitates others in producing animal sounds.

TABLE 3-5 Red flags for sound production.

Be concerned if the child is *not:*	By:
Producing cooing and gooing sounds	6 months
Babbling in repeated sequences of sounds (e.g., baba, gaga)	11 months
Producing 3 different consonant sounds (e.g., b, p, m, n, d, k, t, g, w)	18 months
Imitating any nonspeech sounds (e.g., truck sound, animal sounds)	18 months
Using sound sequences that sound like talking	24 months
Producing (VC)* syllables (e.g., up), (CVC) syllables with a single consonant (e.g., cake), and some vocalizations or words with two or more different consonants (e.g., pat, tummy, bada)	24 months
Producing 6 different consonants	24 months
Producing initial consonants in most words (child says "at" for pat, "ot" for boat)	36 months
Producing 10 different consonants	36 months
Producing any final sounds ("bo" for "boat", "e" for "eat")	36 months

*V = vowel, C = consonant.

The most common early syllable types are Consonant-Vowel (CV) such as "me", VC ("up"), and CVC ("dad") and if CVCV syllables occur, they are typically reduplications (e.g., "wawa" for water). By identifying the types of syllables produced by the child, professionals can make decisions about the child's sound-making capabilities and developmental level. Paul and Jennings (1992) have identified levels of syllable structure expected of young children, such that 24-month-olds should be primarily producing consonant-vowel (CV) syllables, vowel-consonant (VC) syllables, consonant-vowel-consonant (CVC) syllables with a single consonant (e.g., cake), and some vocalizations or words with two or more different consonants (e.g., bada, pat, tummy). As suggested by Paul (1995), the ability to use more than one consonant in an utterance is an important milestone that 24-month-olds with delayed language development have not typically achieved.

Although there is some variability across children, the most frequently used early consonants sounds are *m, n, p, b, d, ch, k, g, h, w, and sh* (Vihman, 1992). The early vowels are typically *a, u,* and *e.* From the work of Paul and Jennings (1992), 18–24 month old typically developing children have been observed to produce an average of 14 different consonants (range, 10–17) in a 10-minute communication sample, whereas 24–36-month-olds use 18 different consonants (range, 15–21).

To help make decisions for referral, there are fairly easy means available to identify the sounds and syllable types the child produces. For young children who do not use word approximations or words, caregiver report and observation of the number and type of sounds the child makes can be compared with what might be expected at the child's chronological age. For young children who are beginning to produce word approximations and some words, parents can be asked to write them down, and professionals can estimate the child's overall number of different consonants and syllable types (e.g., CV, CVC). If the child's sound inventory or type of syllables is quite limited for the child's age and there are other reasons for concern, a referral should be made. Current research has demonstrated that there is a strong relationship between children's sound inventories and their vocabularies. Children who vocalize less than their peers, have limited sound inventories, and have a restricted number of syllable types in both nonverbal vocalizations and meaningful speech, typically have limited vocabularies (Paul & Jennings, 1992; Rescorla & Ratner, 1996). In addition, there are other vocal production behaviors that can be used to identify children who may be at risk for communication deficits. For example, although many children omit some initial consonants ("eep" for "sheep"), omitting *most* or *all* initial consonants in words is not a "typical" behavior that young children display during development; thus, it can be a marker for atypical development. In addition, it is common for young children to omit the final sound in words ("bo" for "boat") and consonants in blends ("bu" for "blue"); however, if there are no final consonants in the speech of a 3-year-old child, there is cause for concern.

Imitation of others can also be a clue into the child's speech production capabilities. Children in the 18–24-month-old range should be readily imitating familiar adults by producing some type of sounds and sound combinations. Common examples include animal sounds, environmental sounds (e.g., truck and train noises), and some speech sounds in play (e.g., "sh" for sleeping babies, "zzz" for bees). Observing the child and asking caregivers for examples of the sounds and syllables the child will imitate can provide an additional look at the young child's sound-making abilities. A continuum of difficulties exists between early sound processing and imitative production and the later appearance of language-learning disabilities (Scarborough, 1990; Stackhouse & Snowling, 1992). Young children who do not learn to imitate speech are those most likely to experience later disabilities in expressive formulation/language organization, developmental apraxia of speech, or language-learning disabilities (Velleman & Strand, 1994). Problems in early imitative ability may include difficulty with sequencing the motor aspects of speech production, limited expressive vocabulary, shortened utterance length, limited sound repertoire, poor syllable structure, and problems in object naming and letter/sound association (Lund & Duchan, 1988; Stackhouse & Snowling, 1992).

When caregivers report that their child age 18–24 months or older avoids imitation of nonspeech (e.g., animal sounds, car sounds) or speech sounds, particularly if the child becomes upset by a caregiver's playful attempts to elicit imitation, the caregivers should be asked about the child's other communication skills. If limitations are noted in these areas, a referral should be made. Anytime unusual sounds are produced frequently by the child (e.g., an abundance of nonspeech sounds added into words, primary use of back of the throat noises); professionals should consider this a factor for recommending further evaluation.

WORD PRODUCTION AND WORD COMBINATIONS

Vocabulary development is an important component of the child's overall development and is critical to both communication development and later academic success. The child's acquisition of new words is impacted not only by his or her sensory and cognitive systems, but also the child's experiences, the input language, and the sociocultural influences that surround the child. Acquisition of the first 50 words is fairly slow, especially compared to the 'vocabulary burst" that frequently occurs after 50 words. Parents who are primarily *middle class*, report their children produce an average of 3.6 words or word-like sounds at 10 months, 11.9 at 12 months, 43.4 at 15 months, 79 by 16 months, 178.9 at 20 months, and 317 by 24 months (Fenson et al., 1993). By these standards, *middle class* children who do not produce 98 words by 24 months of age fall two standard deviations below the mean (placing them in the "at risk" range). Indeed, a traditional red flag for 24 month old children has been the failure to have a production vocabulary of 50 words and/or no two-word combinations (Paul, 1991). However, research has indicated that 10–15% of middle class children have fewer than 50 words at 24 months. Thus, use of this marker as the *only* indicator of delay will produce too many false positives. Indeed, the work of Paul, Looney, and Dahm (1991) has indicated that half of these so-called late talkers by age three will perform at age level on standardized measures. Thus, as suggested by Paul (1991), making a distinction between who will and who will not "outgrow" these early "delays" can be difficult. Although vocabulary size is important, factors such as sound development, social, cognitive, comprehension, play, and imitative skills can also help sort out the "late talkers" from children with language disorders. Thus, an aggregate view across developmental domains in communication and related areas can be a better predictor of later delay.

For identifying emerging words and word approximations, parental report and observation can provide the information around which referral decisions can be made. In this case, identifying the number and type of words or word approximations is useful. As children acquire more words, however, parent report tools such as the *MacArthur Communicative Development Inventories* (MCDI; Fenson et al., 1993) can be used to document production vocabularies up to 30 months of age. The *MacArthur words and gestures* form covers the age range from 9 to 16 months and looks at both production and comprehension vocabularies, as well as gesture use, social games, and pretend play. The 16 to 30 month form (*words and sentences*) does not address comprehension, but does document production vocabulary as well as some aspects of grammar and sentence development. Normative data can then help determine which children are in need of referral, specifically those who fall below the 10th percentile.

Word combinations typically emerge between 18 to 24 months, but not all typically developing children produce word combinations by 24 months (Fenson, et al., 1993). In examining a child's word combinations, the length of the child's utterances can predict the child's overall language development. The typical mean length of utterance is 1.0–1.6 at 18 months, 1.1–2.1 at 21 months, 1.5–2.2 at 24 months, 2.0–3.1 at 30 months, and 2.5–3.9 at 36 months (Miller, 1981). Thus, by 24 months of age, most middle class children are using one to three words per utterance; however, some are just beginning to produce words and have no word combinations (see Table 3–7). Most children begin to combine words when their vocabularies reach between 50 and 100 words. As suggested by many, the correlation between word combinations and vocabulary size is stronger than the correlation between word combinations and age. Thus, vocabulary size should be a helpful marker as to when a child may be expected to begin combining words. Those children with production vocabularies above

TABLE 3-7 Red flags for word productions and word combinations.	
Be concerned if the child is *not:*	**By:**
Producing any words or word approximations	24 months
Producing 50+ words or word approximations	30 months
Producing 100+ words	36 months
Combining words	36 months

100 words who are not combining words, are suspected of communication delays and should be referred for evaluation, especially when they display other risk factors.

CAREGIVER-CHILD INTERACTION

Given the tremendous influence that families have on their child's growth and development, it is prudent for professionals to observe and ask questions about the interactions that the child has with his or her caregivers. There are a variety of means for observing these types of interactions (e.g., use of scales, interviews, observations); however, there are also issues of validity and reliability with each method (see Mahoney, Spiker, & Boyce, 1996 for a thorough review of each method). For example, contextual issues such as the setting (e.g., home, clinic), familiarity of the interactants with the observer(s), type of materials or toys available, type of interaction requested (e.g., completion of particular task, free play), and length of the observation can all affect the ways children and their caregivers interact. Further, sociocultural factors such as culture, ethnicity, and socioeconomic level, as well as personality and interactive style, strongly influence the ways different caregiver-child behaviors are exhibited and viewed. An additional issue in looking at caregiver-child interactions is how to do this in a way that is not critical of the family and keeps the family at the center of the decision-making process reguarding interpretation of different caregiver styles (Crais, 1993; McCollum & Yates, 1994).

One strategy in keeping with family-centered practices is to find out first what things caregivers already do that help the child communicate, and the conditions or situations when the child communicates most effectively. Through this process, family members and professionals can identify skills and strategies that are already used, and identify whether there is a need to make small refinements. There are also a number of behaviors reported in the literature that facilitate communication, including providing responses that are directly related to what the child does/says/looks at, providing positive language models for the child, imitating or expanding the child's actions or words, accepting and reinforcing the child's attempts, and providing the child with adequate time to initiate and respond to adults (Duchan, 1989; Dunst, Lowe, & Bartholomew, 1990). In addition, providing models of desired *communication* behaviors (e.g., gestures, eye gaze, word approximations) can also prove beneficial. These types of behaviors can provide additional suggestions and considerations when observing and talking with caregivers about their interactions with the child. It is clear that most professionals recognize the positive influence that families have on enhancing the communication skills of the child, but few would interpret the family's interaction style as causing or contributing significantly to the child's communication delay. Thus, professionals may need to help parents recognize that they did not cause the child's communication deficit and that it is very likely that what they are doing has facilitated the growth that has taken place. Positive ideas for examining and influencing caregiver-child communicative interactions within a family-centered context can be found in McCollum and Yates (1994).

PROFESSIONAL-CAREGIVER CONSENSUS BUILDING

One difficulty in making decisions about referring a child for evaluation or specialized services is that professionals and caregivers may not always agree that a child needs a referral. Some caregivers have had the experience of relating their concerns about their child to a professional and having the professional either discount their observations entirely or take a "wait and see" approach. Later, some of these caregivers may be quite angry with professionals if their child is found to have difficulties, and they feel that they have lost time in seeking intervention services. Certainly, there are times when a caregiver may underestimate the child's skill level or be concerned about areas that professionals may view as typical for most children. This is particularly true when the child is the caregivers' first and/or only child and they may have limited opportunities for comparing their child with others of the same age. In these instances, further discussion and investigation of the areas highlighted in this chapter may help both the professional and caregivers determine whether a referral is necessary. In addition, recommending additional opportunities for the caregivers to observe other children (e.g., in daycare settings, gymboree classes) may help them identify what are typical or atypical behaviors in their child and others.

At other times, however, *professionals* may believe a child needs referral and the caregivers may not agree. In this instance, the caregivers may even turn away from the professionals because they either do not see the same behaviors or they may not interpret them in the same way as professionals. Historically, in trying to resolve this type of disagreement, professionals may have taken a more directive approach to convince the caregivers that the professionals were "right" and to perhaps "bulldoze" the caregivers into seeking services. In recent years, mounting evidence has accrued to indicate that if early intervention services are to be valued and accepted by caregivers, professionals and caregivers need to gain some type of consensus on the *need* for those services. Indeed, Dunst, Trivette, and Deal (1988) noted that a primary reason for dissatisfaction with early intervention services is the failure of professionals and caregivers to reach consensus on three critical issues: the nature of the presenting concerns, the need for treatment, and the resulting course of action. Clearly, when referral for services is at issue, consensus building is imperative.

In recent years, professionals and caregivers have worked to develop strategies for greater consensus building, and a brief sampling of those strategies is represented here for possible inclusion in professional practices. A common thread across the strategies is the effort on the part of professionals to gain enhanced decision making by caregivers in all aspects of service delivery. One of the best ways to increase decision making is to enhance the role caregivers take in gathering and interpreting information about the child. Rather than professionals gathering all the information, caregivers can be offered the opportunity to be more active in the process. First, caregivers may be given the choice as to what types of information will be used to make decisions about their child. Examples related to identifying concerns about the child include caregivers having the choice to make observations across settings (e.g., home, daycare), gather information from multiple people who interact with the child (e.g., relatives, teachers, other professionals), and utilize multiple sources of information (e.g., observations, interviews, videotapes, parent report tools, or checklists). In addition, caregivers and professionals can decide how best to share the resulting information with each other and others important in the child's life (e.g., phone call, one-to-one meeting, meeting with whole family and/or other professionals). Increasingly, the literature indicates that when caregivers are more active in the information-gathering process, there is a greater basis for discussion between professionals and caregivers, caregivers become better observers of their child's behavior, and there is a greater synthesis between the views of caregivers and professionals (Bloch & Seitz, 1989; Dinnebeil & Rule, 1994). Clearly, caregivers have information to share that is typically unavailable to professionals because they are able to observe larger samples of behaviors in naturalistic environments; thus, their input can enhance the validity and reliability of the early decision-making process (Simeonsson, Edmondson, Smith, Carnahan, & Bucy, 1995; Squires, Nickel, & Bricker, 1990). Further, the predictability of the screening process has been shown to increase with the combination of professional administered and caregiver completed measures (Henderson & Meisels, 1994). Thus, professionals may want to consider a variety of options available to caregivers in coming to the important decision of making a referral for evaluation and early intervention services.

SUMMARY

For all children who have or who may be at risk for communication deficits, professionals and caregivers need to work together to form the "village" that surrounds the child to help identify possible difficulties. In working within a collaborative approach where caregivers are active decision makers, professionals and caregivers can utilize the strategies identified to determine whether a child is in need of a referral for evaluation for suspected communication difficulties. In addition, in becoming more aware of the many interconnections between communication development and related domains, professionals and caregivers may intervene earlier when there are suspected communication deficits.

REFERENCES

Bloch, J. S., & Seitz, M. (1989). Parents as assessors of children. *Social Work in Education, 11,* 226–244.

Carpenter, M., Nagell, K., & Tomasello, M. (1998). Social cognition, joint attention, and communicative competence from 9 to 15 months of age. *Monographs of the Society for Research in Child Development, 63(4),* Serial #255, 1–175.

Chapman, R. (1978). Comprehension strategies in children. In J. Kavanaugh & W. Strange (Eds.), *Speech and language in the laboratory, school, and clinic* (pp. 308–327. Cambridge, MA: MIT Press.

Crais, E. (1993). Families and professionals as collaborators in assessment. *Topics in Language Disorders, 14(1),* 29–40.

Dinnebeil, L., & Rule, S. (1994). Congruence between parents' and professionals' judgments about the development of young children with disabilities: A review of the literature. *Topics in Early Childhood Special Education, 14(1),* 1–25.

Duchan, J. (1989). Evaluating adults' talk to children: Addressing adult attunement. *Seminars in Speech and Language, 10,* 17–27.

Dunst, C., Lowe, L., & Bartholomew, P. (1990). Contingent social responsiveness, family ecology, and infant communicative competence. *National Student Speech-Language-Hearing Journal, 17,* 39–49.

Dunst, C., Trivette, C., & Deal, A. (1988). *Enabling and empowering families.* Cambridge, MA: Brookline Books.

Eilers, R., & Oller, K. (1994). Infants and the early diagnosis of severe hearing impairment. *Journal of Pediatrics, 124,* 199–203.

Fenson, L., Dale, P., Reznick, S., Thal, D., Bates, E., Hartung, J., Pethick, S., & Reilly, J. (1993). *MacArthur communicative development inventories.* San Diego, CA: Singular Publishing Group.

Henderson, L., & Meisels, S. (1994). Parental involvement in the developmental screening of their young child: A multiple-source perspective. *Journal of Early Intervention, 18(2),* 141–154.

Lund, N., & Duchan, J. (1988). *Assessing children's language in naturalistic contexts.* Englewood, NJ: Prentice Hall.

Mahoney, G., Spiker, D., & Boyce, G. (1996). Clinical assessments of parent-child interactions: Are professionals ready to implement this practice? *Topics in Early Childhood Special Education, 16(1),* 26–50.

McCollum, J., & Yates, T. (1994). Dyad as focus, triad as means: A family-centered approach to supporting parent-child interactions. *Infants and Young Children, 6(4),* 54–63.

Miller, J. (1981). *Assessing language production in children.* Baltimore, MD: University Park Press.

Paul, R. (1991). Profiles of toddlers with slow expressive language development. *Topics in Language Disorders, 11(4),* 1–13.

Paul, R. (1995). *Language disorders from infancy through adolescence.* St. Louis, MO: Mosby.

Paul, R., & Jennings, P. (1992). Phonological behavior in toddlers with slow expressive language development. *Journal of Speech and Hearing Research, 35,* 99–107.

Paul, R., Looney, S., & Dahm, P. (1991). Communication and socialization skills at ages 2 and 3 in "late talking" young children. *Journal of Speech and Hearing Disorders, 34,* 858–865.

Rescorla, L., & Ratner, N. (1996). Phonetic profiles of toddlers with expressive language impairment (SLI-E). *Journal of Speech and Hearing Research, 39,* 153–165.

Scarborough, H.S. (1990). Very early language deficits in dyslexic children. *Child Development, 61,* 1728–1743.

Simeonsson, R., Edmondson, R., Smith, T., Carnahan, S., & Bucy, J. (1995). Family involvement in multidisciplinary team evaluation: Professional and parent perspectives. *Childcare, Health, and Development, 21(3),* 199–215.

Smith, A., Goffman, L., & Stark, R. (1995). Speech motor development. *Seminars in Speech and Language, 16(2),* 87–99.

Squires, J. K., Nickel, R., & Bricker, D. (1990). Use of parent-completed developmental questionnaires for child find and screening. *Infants and Young Children, 3,* 46–57.

Stackhouse, J., & Snowling, M. (1992). Barriers to literacy development in two cases of developmental verbal dyspraxia: A longitudinal study. *European Journal of Communication Disorders, 27,* 35–54.

U.S. Department of Education. (1996). *Eighteenth Annual Report to Congress on the Implementation of the Individuals with Disabilities Education Act.* Division of Innovation and Development, Office of Special Education Programs. Washington, D.C.

Velleman, S., & Strand, E. (1994). Developmental verbal dyspraxia. In J. Bernthal & N. Bankson (Eds.), *Child phonology: characteristics, assessment, and intervention with special populations,* pp. 110–139. NY: Thieme Medical Publishers.

Vihman, M. (1992). Early syllables and the construction of phonology. In C. Ferguson, L. Menn, & C. Stoel-Gammon (Eds.), *Phonological development: Models, research, implications,* pp. 393–422. Timonium, MD: York Press.

Wetherby, A., Cain, D., Yonclass, D., & Walker, V. (1988). Analysis of intentional communication of normal children from the prelinguistic to the multiword stage. *Journal of Speech and Hearing Research, 31,* 240–252.

Wetherby, A., & Prizant, B. (1993). *Communication and symbolic behavior scales.* Chicago: Riverside Press.

Part II: Models for Planning and Implementation

INTRODUCTION

Part II of this text features a description of several outstanding programs in the United States, as depicted by the clinicians responsible for those programs. It should be noted that many screening programs combine two or more of the technologies described here. For example, some infant hearing screening programs have adopted a two-step screening procedure that employs otoacoustic emissions as a first-level screen followed by automated auditory brainstem responses for infants who do not pass the otoacoustic emissions. The models described here are by no means exhaustive. Those responsible for planning and implementing a program must adapt their procedures and protocols to the goals of the screening program and individual circumstances unique to each setting.

The Colorado Newborn Hearing Screening Project: Steps for Developing New Programs

CHAPTER 4

Deborah Hayes, Ph.D.
and Vickie Thomson, M.A.

INTRODUCTION

Development and implementation of a successful screening program proceeds from careful planning. Before making any decisions regarding screening method, technology, or even target population, a Screening Program Manager must be identified and an Advisory Committee assembled. These key screening program participants define screening program goals and outcome expectations and identify potential obstacles to program success. In most cases, the Screening Program Manager is a licensed audiologist who will be responsible for program design, implementation, and evaluation. The Advisory Committee participants include hospital or school administrators, physicians, nurses, teachers, and parents. Because screening for hearing loss or middle ear effusion in some populations remains controversial (Bess and Paradise, 1992; Paradise, 1999), all program participants should be well-informed about the rationale for the proposed screening program and the benefits to children, families, and the community.

Several investigators have described well-designed hearing screening programs, especially universal newborn hearing screening programs (UNHS). These investigators have highlighted important components of program development such as stakeholder involvement, role definition, individualized program design, short- and long-term plans and goals, quality control, and quality assurance and risk management. As discussed below, each of these elements contributes to overall program success.

Marlowe (1993) was among the first to describe development and implementation of a universal newborn hearing-screening program at a private, not-for-profit community hospital. In designing the program, Marlowe noted the importance of meeting with representatives of all disciplines who would be impacted by implementation of UNHS, including hospital administration, medical staff, nursing, volunteers/hospital auxiliary, and development/marketing personnel. In addition to describing the benefits of hearing screening for infants and families, she stressed the importance of identifying and documenting the benefits of UNHS for each affected group. For physicians attending in the nursery, for example, Marlowe noted that the UNHS program provided state-of-the-art care for its patients and enhanced its liability protection. Marlowe highlights the importance of identifying and involving key stakeholders in the first steps of planning a screening program.

103

Johnson and her colleagues (1993) describe the implementation of an UNHS research protocol at Women and Infants Hospital of Rhode Island. This important project, the Rhode Island Hearing Assessment Project (RIHAP), demonstrated the feasibility of UNHS at a major teaching hospital with more than 9000 deliveries per year, which includes both well-baby and neonatal intensive care populations. Johnson and her colleagues stress the importance of identifying the specific responsibilities of program participants, from screening technician to medical director. Precise definition of roles and responsibilities for each program participant is a critical success factor for any screening program.

Roush (1990) describes the various factors that must be considered in planning, implementing, and evaluating an audiologic screening program. Roush suggests examination of the underlying rationale for screening as a necessary first step in designing audiologic screening programs to detect hearing loss and middle ear disease in preschool and school age children. He also notes the importance of factors such as test environment, instrumentation, screening personnel, record keeping and follow-up in any screening program. Rather than describing a single screening protocol for all settings, Roush encourages individualized program design to meet the unique needs and goals of the screening program.

In describing a statewide system for UNHS, Thomson (1997) described the roles of an Advisory Board and an audiology coordinator in designing and implementing an overall short- and long-term plan. Initially, the Colorado statewide program was voluntary; that is, individual hospitals were approached to add newborn hearing screening as a service component of routine newborn care. The audiology coordinator, sponsored by the state department of health, was essential for providing support and facilitating development of a program in each hospital. In addition, with the assistance of an Advisory Committee, the audiology coordinator developed a statewide five-year plan that included quantifiable benchmarks (e.g., number of hospitals screening), and community education components. Table 4–1 summarizes the Colorado Newborn Hearing Screening Project 5-Year Plan. As shown in the table, the plan addresses identification of potential screening sites, data collection and management, and opportunities for professional and public education. Thomson underscores the importance of developing a systematic, planned approach to screening program development and the roles of multiple stakeholders in implementing the plan.

Albright and Finitzo (1997) provide valuable insight into development of quality control in hearing screening programs. These investigators identified and defined critical quality indicators that they monitored in newborn hearing screening programs. Albright and Finitzo stress the importance of operational definitions of quality indicators so that key stakeholders agree on meaning. In addition, they demonstrate how quality indicators permit ongoing quality assessment and program evaluation.

In concert with issues of quality assurance, issues of risk management should be addressed in development of any screening program (Marlowe, 1997; Tharpe and Clayton, 1997). Audiologic screening programs must be designed with careful attention to legal, equipment, and documentation issues. Legal issues may include requirement for informed consent or permission, and ensuring compliance with the accepted standard of care. In addition, practitioner licensure and program supervision should be addressed during program devel-

TABLE 4-1   Colorado Newborn Hearing Screening Project 5-Year Plan.

Year I:

- Contact 10–20 major birthing hospitals.
- Implement universal newborn hearing screening in 3 hospitals.
- Educate professionals (audiologists, neonatologists, nurses, pediatricians, and family physicians) about the goals of the Colorado Project.

Year II:

- Implement data collection system.
- Expand universal newborn hearing screening to 10 hospitals.
- Convene monthly informational meetings for audiologists managing screening programs and other interested professionals.

Year III:

- Analyze screening and diagnosis results for years I and II.
- Expand universal newborn hearing screening to 10 additional hospitals, including rural hospitals.
- Provide presentations at national meetings and workshops.

Year IV:

- Expand universal newborn hearing screening to remaining interested or targeted hospitals.
- Support and sustain existing programs.
- Promote public awareness of the importance of early identification and intervention of hearing loss.

Year V:

- Promote legislation for universal newborn hearing screening.
- Support development of local advisory boards and regional hearing coordinators.
- Disseminate information about Colorado Project through professional and public media publications.
- Implement a computerized data management system.

opment. Equipment issues include appropriate and approved use of medical devices. Documentation issues include prompt notification of screening results only to those individuals legally entitled to receive this information. As noted by the Joint Committee on Infant Hearing (2000), infant and family rights and confidentiality of information must be addressed in UNHS programs.

As these and other investigators report, many aspects of program design, implementation, and evaluation must be considered prior to implementing any screening program. Before convening the first planning meeting, the Screening Program Manager should take three important steps. First, the Screening Program Manager should prepare an outline of the various topics to be addressed. As described below ("Designing a Successful Screening Program"), topics such as 1) defining program rationale, 2) identifying potential barriers to success, and 3) describing program benchmarks and quality indicators are just three of many topics that must be discussed before program implementation. Second, the Screening Program Manager should complete a literature search of relevant clinical and research literature. Reports provided by colleagues who have implemented audiologic screening programs frequently contain valuable information for addressing universal and/or local barriers to success. Finally, the Screening Program Manager should collect relevant guidelines on the proposed screening activity. State departments of health, national professional organizations, and/or multidisciplinary committees such as the Joint Committee on Infant Hearing often produce position papers or guidelines that can assist in developing screening programs using currently validated procedures. With these three steps completed, the Screening Program Manager is then ready to convene the first planning meeting.

DESIGNING A SUCCESSFUL SCREENING PROGRAM

Many elements contribute to a successful screening program. In all cases, successful programs begin with a planning process that addresses, at a minimum, the following considerations:

1. What is the rationale for the proposed screening program?
2. What are the potential barriers to a successful screening program?
3. How will the program be evaluated? What are accepted or reasonable benchmarks and quality indicators for this screening activity?
4. What referral and follow-up strategies can be effectively implemented to ensure appropriate outcomes for children and families?
5. How will parents be informed about the screening process?
6. How will the screening protocol be implemented (e.g., selecting the screening technology, screening environment, identifying the screening personnel and their training needs, and developing a data management system to monitor program outcomes)?
7. How will the community be educated about the value of audiologic screening of infants and children?

Defining the Rationale for the Proposed Screening Program

It is critically important that the Screening Program Manager, the Advisory Committee, and all program participants understand the rationale for the proposed screening program. In the case of audiologic screening of infants and children, the rationale for early detection and treatment of hearing loss is sound and generally well accepted. Numerous authors have examined the rationale for universal newborn hearing screening relative to the justification for screening (e.g., prevalence of hearing loss, consequences of undetected hearing loss, ability to detect hearing loss before it is clinically evident, utility of early detection and intervention in improving outcome, and cost effectiveness). In their recent position statement on newborn and infant hearing loss, the American Academy of Pediatrics (1999) states that the minimum criteria necessary to justifying universal screening are achievable by effective universal newborn hearing screening programs. One useful approach for examining the rationale for the proposed

TABLE 4-2 Criteria for justifying and evidence for supporting universal newborn hearing screening.

Selected criteria needed to justify screening	Results relative to hearing loss
Prevalence of disorder	3 per 1,000 newborns*
Age of detection in absence of screening	14 months or older**
Consequences of undetected disorder	Language delay; academic failure***
Availability of diagnosis and intervention	Federal and state mandates (i.e., Medicaid EPSDT; Part C)
Cost per case detected	~ $9,600****

*Finitzo, Albright, and O'Neal, 1998.
**Elssman, Matkin, and Sabo, 1987; Harrison and Roush, 1996.
***Yoshinago-Itano, Sedey, Coulter, and Mehl, 1998; Carney and Moeller, 1998.
****Mehl and Thomson, 1998.

screening program is to develop a list of justifying criteria similar to that shown in Table 4-2. As shown in Table 4-2, each justifying criterion should be addressed and supporting research and clinical studies should be cited. Whatever the proposed screening program, examining the rationale relative to various justifying criteria is a worthwhile exercise. Additional justifying criteria that can be examined include sensitivity and specificity of the proposed screening technique and cost per screening test.

Identifying Potential Barriers to Success

The Screening Program Manager and Advisory Committee should also closely examine potential barriers to a successful screening program. Barriers to screening program success may range from lack of institutional support for capital equipment and personnel to active opposition from key stakeholders such as parents, physicians, or other professionals. In many instances, barriers arise from lack of program "buy-in" by key stakeholders; in the examples above, key stakeholders include institutional officials (e.g., hospital or school administrators) as well as parents, physicians, and other professionals. The Screening Program Manager should make every attempt to identify and involve the key stakeholders from the onset of program planning and to address objections to the proposed program before program implementation. Even program facility barriers, such as an inadequate or inappropriate screening environment, may be overcome if the key stakeholder in control of facilities is included in early program planning.

Evaluating Program Effectiveness; Defining Benchmarks and Quality Indicators

Prior to designing the screening program, the Screening Program Manager and Advisory Committee should define how program effectiveness will be measured. Currently accepted benchmarks, quality indicators, and monitoring protocols for the proposed screening activity should be reviewed and adopted as appropriate. In the Joint Committee on Infant Hearing 2000 Position Statement, benchmarks are defined as, "quantifiable goals or targets by which a…program may be monitored and evaluated…" Quality indicators "reflect a result in relation to a stated benchmark…" Monitoring protocols are simply those techniques employed to collect, analyze, and review quality data in a timely and consistent manner. The JCIH recommends several benchmarks for UNHS such as 1) hospitals or birthing centers screen at least 95% of infants during their birth admission or before one month of age, 2) the referral rate for audiologic and medical evaluation following the screening process should be 4% or less, and 3) at least 70% of infants who fail hearing screening return for follow-up. Whenever possible, benchmarks should be based on research or clinical studies and defined prior to program implementation. Once a screening program is implemented, quality indicators should be monitored on a regular basis to assess program achievement relative to the stated benchmark. Any deviation in program achievement, for example, failing an unexpectedly large number of children or recording a substantial increase in loss to follow-up, should result in prompt investigation and institution of corrective actions.

Developing Referral and Follow-Up Strategies

The Screening Program Manager and Advisory Committee should identify appropriate referral and follow-up strategies to ensure adequate return for follow-up and screening outcome. The first step is to include those individuals or agencies that will be responsible for assuring follow-up. In a hospital newborn hearing screening program, for example, physicians, audiologists, Part C coordinators, nursery staff, parent consumers and early interventionists are part of the team that develops a follow-up protocol. It is very important that families and those responsible for follow-up have a clear picture of what steps need to be taken when an infant or child does not pass the screening. Screening without appropriate follow-up will not provide the desired outcome.

When developing a follow-up protocol from screening, the questions that need to be addressed are:

How will parents receive the screening results?

Parents have the right to be informed as soon as possible of the screening results so that immediate intervention can take place. One of the most troublesome aspects of any screening program is the poor return for follow-up. Two approaches may improve the percentage of families who follow through with the recommendations. First, giving parents information on the screening results and having clear, direct recommendations will assist with follow-up efforts. Second, providing the information in the parents' native language, written and verbally if necessary, will help assure that parents understand the recommendations for follow-up.

Who will be responsible for assuring the family follows through with the recommendations?

Clearly defining professional and agency roles in the follow-up process will identify the party responsible for ensuring each infant and child's follow-up. This process is critical to also ensuring that parents return for follow-up.

Who will be responsible for notifying the parents, professionals, and various agencies of the results?

The individual or agency responsible for notifying parents, other professionals, and agencies entitled to receive screening results must be identified. In the case of newborn hearing screening, it may be necessary to inform parents, the primary care physician, medical records, the state department of health, and early intervention agencies of screening results. Informed consent and release of information must be addressed in defining this aspect of the screening program.

What is the next step following screening?

This will depend on the type of hearing screening program being implemented and the outcome of the screen. In most hearing screening programs the child is rescreened within several weeks after the initial screen to decrease the number of referrals for more expensive medical or audiologic diagnostic evaluations. In the preschool or school-age populations, referral to the primary care physician or medical home may be warranted to rule out middle ear fluid or to remove debris in the ear canal.

How will infants and children who are at risk for acquired or progressive hearing loss, regardless of the screening outcome, continue to be monitored for hearing loss?

Parents should be given appropriate speech and language milestone information so they can monitor their child's development. They should be educated and encouraged to contact an audiologist any time they have concerns about their child's hearing. Parents, physicians, and other care providers should be reminded that passing a hearing screening does not guarantee normal hearing in the future.

Informing Parents of the Screening Process

Parents are important participants in the screening process. Informed parent consent or permission, confidentiality, and notification of results are issues that need to be addressed by the Screening Program Manager and Advisory Committee. Parents should understand the value of audiologic screening for their child and the importance of follow through with recommendations.

Assuring that "informed consent" is obtained as part of the screening program will give parents the opportunity to become educated about and participate in their child's screening. States may have mandates that govern the rules around "informed consents." Acceptable informed consent may range from verbal consent and provision of written information with an "opt-out" requirement, to a formal signed consent.

Written materials are essential educational tools that also provide parents with further recommendations or referral information. Brochures or information sheets should include a simple description of the technology/technique for audiologic screening and what recommendations will be made if a child does not pass the screening. Parents should understand that screening is a technique to identify those infants or children at risk for hearing loss and/or middle ear dysfunction, and that the consequences of not complying with the recommendations for follow-up can result in delayed speech, language, and other developmental problems. Many state departments of health and education have parent-oriented literature on hearing screening, hearing, speech and language development, or developmental milestones that can be helpful in a hearing screening program.

Confidentiality of the screening results is important in any screening program. The parents must sign a release of information if the results are going to be shared with other professionals or state agencies. During the "informed consent" process parents may sign a form that not only grants permission for the agency to perform the screen, but also allows for the results to be reported to various individuals or agencies. In some state newborn hearing screening programs, the results may be given to the primary care physician and the department of health for tracking and follow-up.

The standard of care for the screening program may dictate how parents are informed of their child's screening results. In newborn hearing screening programs, it is preferable to give the parents the results of the hearing screening prior to hospital discharge. This allows the family to ask questions and immediately schedule a rescreening if necessary. Informing parents in a timely manner, and providing clear, concise recommendations and referral information may prevent unnecessary parental stress or concerns.

Planning Screening Program Implementation

Screening Equipment

Multiple commercial devices are typically available to perform the desired screening test (i.e., infant hearing screening, middle ear screening). The technology selected should provide the highest specificity (will pass unaffected individuals) and the highest sensitivity (will identify hearing loss or middle ear dysfunction). In newborn hearing screening programs, two objective technologies are used, otoacoustic emissions and auditory brainstem response as discussed elsewhere in this book.

Regardless of the screening technology selected, equipment must have routine calibration and safety checks. Training in equipment calibration and troubleshooting techniques is important for reducing screening error.

Screening Environment

Screening for hearing loss or middle ear dysfunction requires a quiet test environment. The Screening Program Manager should evaluate the proposed screening environment to assess variables that might affect screening outcome, such as ambient noise level, electrical interference, and visual distractions. If parents will be attending the screening, as in newborn hearing screening programs, there should be adequate room and comfortable seating for the family. Neonatal Intensive Care Units (NICU) have additional precautions and the screeners should work closely with nursing personnel to determine the appropriate time, location, and conditions for screening. When screening older children, a room with fewer distractions is recommended so the child can easily attend to the task at hand.

Screening Personnel

Selection of the appropriate personnel for screening programs will depend on the population being screened and the equipment selected (e.g., infant screening using automated brainstem technologies requires good manual dexterity and good vision to utilize the electrode montage). Advances in automated screening technologies permit the use of support personnel to provide the screening in many programs.

Some states have regulations within the audiology licensure laws that define and limit the use of support personnel for screening purposes. Health and education institutions may also have specific guidelines for use of support personnel. Support personnel may be required to attend classes to receive certification on their competency skills. If support personnel are used to perform the screening procedure, each screener should complete a "Competency Based Orientation" to the screening program rationale, goals, and expectations, an example of which is shown below.

Competency Based Orientation for a Newborn Hearing Screener:

1. Demonstrates responsibility as a screener for the Newborn Hearing Screening Program:
   A. Complies with the policies outlined in the Newborn Hearing Screening Manual.
   B. Maintains confidentiality of all patient information.
   C. Initiates the preparation steps for screening upon arrival in the nursery; obtains the daily census and identifies which infants need to be screened.
   D. Notifies the audiologist if there are any concerns about the equipment.
2. Demonstrates excellent communication skills with the family and staff:
   A. Obtains verbal permission from the family and explains the newborn hearing screening procedure.
   B. Obtains a signed waiver if family refuses to have the screen.
   C. Records and files the screening results in the baby's medical record chart and places a copy in the physician's hospital mailbox.
3. Demonstrates skill in administering a safe and reliable hearing screening test; prepares the infant for screening by:
   A. Appropriate electrode placement and attachment of correct cable leads.
   B. Positioning ear couplers appropriately.
   C. Making sure that the infant is in the position recommended by nursing to prevent choking.
   D. Following troubleshooting guidelines.

Educating, training, and evaluating screening personnel are critical to program success. Screeners should understand the importance of early identification and intervention of hearing loss. A licensed audiologist should directly supervise screening personnel during initial training stages to ensure appropriate use, maintenance, and calibration of screening equipment. The screener should also be able to demonstrate skills in working with infants or children, and knowledge of infection control including universal precautions.

Managing Data

Tracking infants and children through the follow-up process is necessary for documenting the efficacy of the screening program. Administrators need data to demonstrate that the screening program is providing the outcome of early identification and intervention. Monitoring quality indicators on a regular basis (monthly or quarterly) will allow the Screening Program Manager to assess program outcome relative to established benchmarks, to identify problem areas, and to redefine policies, procedures, and protocols. Benchmarks recommended for some aspects of UNHS programs include (American Academy of Pediatrics, 1999; Joint Committee on Infant Hearing, 2000):

Data Item	*Benchmark*
1. The number of infants born.	
2. The number of infants screened.	95%
3. The number of infants referred (or did not pass the screen at discharge).	<4%
4. The number of infants who returned for a rescreen.	>70%
5. The number of infants who were referred to an audiologist.	<1%
6. The number of infants who were confirmed with a hearing loss.	

Computerized data management systems are the most efficient tool for tracking data items. Manual systems are difficult to maintain, burdensome, and prone to loss and error. Depending on the screening technology, automated data management systems may be available in an associated software package.

Educating the Community on the Importance of Audiologic Screening for Infants and Children

There are multiple audiences who have special informational needs. Parents, other professionals, such as school or hospital administrators, physicians, and intervention programs, agencies, service organizations, and the general public should all receive information regarding the proposed screening program. The professionals and agencies responsible for assuring the system need to understand the importance of audiologic screening and their specific role in the follow-up process. In newborn hearing screening programs several individuals may be responsible for the follow-up from screening through intervention. For example, the screening coordinator will schedule the follow-up rescreen, the physician will assure the referral to the diagnostic audiologist, and the audiologist will refer directly to an early intervention program. Each of these individuals may also be required to submit documentation to various agencies such as Part C or Departments of Health. These agencies may also report information to federal agencies such as the Centers for Disease Control and Prevention, for surveillance data collection.

Professional organizations can provide expertise and financial assistance for educational efforts to the general public and other professionals. For example, the American Academy of Audiology and the American Speech, Language and Hearing Association offer a variety of materials at little or no cost to their members and the general public. Materials include high-quality, professionally produced public service announcements for use in local public broadcast and print media. Local grocery stores and other vendors may permit program announcements on grocery bags or in storefront windows.

In many communities, organizations such as Lions Club, Sertoma, United Way, March of Dimes, and Quota Club may be approached to assist with the screening program. These service clubs may provide funding for equipment, supplies, or educational materials. Members of these community service organizations may also assist in developing a public awareness campaign.

SUMMARY

Without a doubt, development of successful audiologic screening programs is one of the most challenging aspects of current clinical practice. Many factors must be considered before a single infant or child is screened. In the preceding discussion, we intentionally listed "Planning Screening Program Implementation" as among the last issues for the screening program participants to address. Issues such as referral and follow-up strategies, program evaluation, and parent and community involvement must be addressed before any screening program is designed.

The current literature contains numerous reports of development and implementation of successful audiologic screening programs. A feature common to these programs is the careful program pre-planning, followed by systematic collection of relevant data to demonstrate program effectiveness. The reports cited in this chapter highlight some additional features of program design that can be incorporated into any audiologic screening program.

Every audiologic screening program must be designed to result in improved hearing outcomes for children. Early identification and intervention should drive every aspect of program design, and every program should achieve this goal. Although technological advances will certainly improve audiologic screening in the future, the demonstrated outcome must remain better hearing for infants and children.

REFERENCES

Albright, K., & Finitzo, T. (1997). Texas hospitals' quality control approach to universal infant hearing detection. *American Journal of Audiology, 6*, 88–90.

American Academy of Pediatrics, Task Force on Newborn and Infant Hearing. (1999). Newborn and infant hearing loss: detection and intervention. *Pediatrics, 103*, 527–530.

Bess, F. H. and Paradise, J. L. (1992). Universal screening for infant hearing: Not simple, not risk-free, not necessarily beneficial, and not presently justified. *Pediatrics, 98*, 330–334.

Carney, A. E., & Moeller, M. P. (1998). Treatment efficacy: hearing loss in children. *Journal of Speech-Language-Hearing Research, 41*, S61–S84.

Elssman, S. A., Matkin, N. D., & Sabo, M. P. (1987). Early identification of congenital sensorineural hearing impairment. *The Hearing Journal, 12*, 191–198.

Finitzo, T., Albright, K., & O'Neal, J. (1998). The newborn with hearing loss: detection in the nursery. *Pediatrics, 102*, 1452–1460.

Harrison, M., & Roush, J. (1996). Age of suspicion, identification and intervention for infant and young children with hearing loss: A national study. *Ear and Hearing, 17*, 55–62.

Johnson, M. J., Maxon, A. B., White, K. R., & Vohr, B. R. (1993). Operating a hospital-based universal newborn hearing screening program using transient evoked otoacoustic emissions. In *Seminars in Hearing*, K. R. White, & T. R. Behrens, (Eds.), *The Rhode Island Hearing Assessment Project: Implications for Universal Newborn Hearing Screening, 14*, 46–56.

Joint Committee on Infant Hearing. 2000 Position Statement. *Audiology Today*, in press.

Marlowe, J. A. (1993). Screening all newborns for hearing impairment in a community hospital. *American Journal of Audiology, 2*, 22–25.

Marlowe, J. A. (1997). The risk management perspective of the universal detection of hearing loss in newborns. *American Journal of Audiology, 6*, 100–102.

Mehl, A. L., & Thomson, V. (1998). Newborn hearing screening: The great omission. *Pediatrics*, 4th ed.

Paradise, J. L. (1999). Universal newborn hearing screening: Should we leap before we look? *Pediatrics, 103*, 670–672.

Roush, J. (1990). Identification of hearing loss and middle ear disease in preschool and school-age children. In *Seminars in Hearing*, A. O. Diefendorf, (Ed.), *Pediatric Audiology, 11*, 357–371.

Tharpe, A. M., & Clayton, E. W. (1997). Newborn hearing screening: Issues in legal liability and quality assurance. *American Journal of Audiology, 6*, 5–12.

Thomson, V. (1997). The Colorado newborn hearing screening project. *American Journal of Audiology, 6*, 74–77.

Yoshinaga-Itano, C., Sedey, A., Coulter, D. K., & Mehl, A. L. (1998). Language of early and later identified children with hearing loss. *Pediatrics, 102*, 1161–1171.

Acknowledgment: Preparation of this chapter was supported in part by grants from the Maternal Child Health Bureau (6 MCJ-08NH022; 2-T73-MC-00011–04).

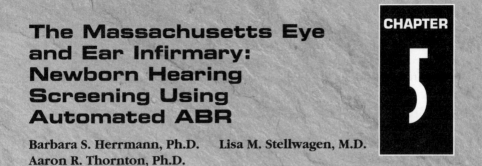

The Massachusetts Eye and Ear Infirmary: Newborn Hearing Screening Using Automated ABR

CHAPTER 5

Barbara S. Herrmann, Ph.D.   Lisa M. Stellwagen, M.D.
Aaron R. Thornton, Ph.D.

GOALS OF THE SCREENING PROGRAM

The newborn hearing screening program at the Massachusetts General Hospital (MGH) began in 1981 out of a concern of the MGH nursery staff regarding the high incidence of hearing loss in their Neonatal Intensive Care Unit (NICU) graduates. From the beginning of the screening program in the NICU through its expansion into the well-baby nursery in 1997, the goal has been to identify newborns having sufficient hearing loss to delay the development of speech and language, and to get those babies appropriate intervention within one month of screening. Our success in reaching this goal depends upon our success in attaining two procedural goals. The first goal is to screen each admitted newborn infant before discharge to either the baby's home or the hospital of birth. The second is to complete an auditory-evoked response threshold evaluation either before discharge or within a week of discharge for every baby failing both ears in the screening.

SETTING

The Massachusetts General Hospital is an 844-bed general hospital affiliated with the Harvard Medical School. From the late 1950s to 1994, the MGH Neonatology Department consisted only of a Level 3, tertiary neonatal intensive care nursery. In 1994, a complete maternity service with associated Level 1 (well-baby) and Level 2 (special care) nurseries were opened as the MGH Mother and Child Center in a new building in the MGH complex. The Level 3 nursery is on the third floor of the new building, while the Level 1 and Level 2 nurseries are on the thirteenth floor. The Labor and Delivery Unit is on the fourteenth floor.

Newborn hearing screening began in the MGH Level 3 nursery in 1981 in partnership with the Audiology Department of the Massachusetts Eye and Ear Infirmary. The Massachusetts Eye and Ear Infirmary (MEEI) is a Harvard-affiliated specialty hospital for treatment of eye and ear, nose and throat disorders. The Audiology Department is large with 23 audiologists on staff and a yearly patient census of approximately 15,000. The department provides a full range of audiologic services, including standard audiometric evaluations, auditory-evoked response evaluations (AERs), hearing aid dispensing, facial nerve evaluation, and OR monitoring. While MEEI is an independently chartered hospital, it is physically attached to MGH via a shared connecting building. The Audiology Department occupies part of the second floor of the Infirmary, which connects with the third floor of the MGH Ellison Building and the Level 3 nursery.

TARGET POPULATION

All newborns admitted to the Level 1, 2, or 3 nurseries are screened for hearing loss. The census of the Level 3 nursery fluctuates between 250 and 350 babies per year. The census of the Level 1 nursery is approximately 2,200 births. Hearing screening has always been a standing nursery order eliminating the need for individual orders by each baby's primary physician. We have always used a standing order for screening because it eliminates paperwork and conversation, and results in a more consistent and efficient screening service.

SCREENING PERSONNEL

Babies are screened by audiologists from the Audiology Department of MEEI. In 1981, we began by bringing the NICU infants over to the sound-treated environment of the Auditory-Evoked Response Laboratory at MEEI. At that time, the sophistication of evoked response equipment and the need to explore the robustness of the auditory brainstem response in babies prompted us to screen in a controlled environment with the goal of transferring the screening to the nursery when the targeted performance could be established in the NICU. During this time, screening was done by very experienced audiologists who specialized in evoked potential procedures. When an intelligent, automated, and portable infant hearing screening instrument became available in 1984, we transferred the screening to the nursery. With the automated instrument, we were able to change the screening personnel to less-experienced audiologists and maintain the same program performance (Herrmann, Thornton, & Joseph, 1995).

When the screening program was expanded to include the Level 1 and Level 2 nurseries, we continued to use audiologists as screeners. At present, the screening personnel requirements are still less than a full-time employee. An audiologist is more useful to the department during non-screening hours than a technician trained specifically for newborn hearing screening. Since we have a large audiology staff, backup for sickness, vacation, and other absences are more effectively managed when the entire staff is familiar with the screening procedures. Because the automated screener does not require knowledge of audiology nor experience with evoked response for consistent results, newborn hearing screening is one of the first procedures learned by new staff. Weekends are covered by the audiologist on call, who is given compensatory time the next week.

INSTRUMENTATION

The choice of a screening method is often controversial. Although we had developed an automated method for screening babies in 1978–1979 (Thornton, 1978; Sprague & Thornton; 1979; Thornton & Obenour, 1981), there was no effective infant hearing screener commercially available when we began the screening program in 1981. We began evaluating the ABR for infant hearing screening, which led to the development of the ALGO I Infant Hearing Screener (Natus Medical Inc.) (Herrmann et al., 1995). During this development, we targeted several requirements for an infant hearing screening method. First, the method should have as close to a 100% hit rate as possible. This requirement was important because passing a deaf baby gives a false sense of security, and delays the identification of that child more than if the baby had never been screened at all.

Second, the screening method should have a low false positive rate on the initial screen. The false positive rate is reflected in the overall referral rate of a screening program. Since the incidence of newborn hearing loss is essentially the same across nurseries, the higher the referral rate, the higher the false positive rate. The false positive rate needs to be low to keep costs under control. It is also important for keeping the anxiety of parents and the nuisance to the primary physician at a minimum. High false positive rates desensitize physicians to the importance and urgency of follow-up. Figure 5–1 illustrates how following and evaluating false positives are a large part of the overall cost of newborn hearing screening.

In this figure, the costs of two screening programs are compared, one with a referral rate of 10% and another with a referral rate of 1%. The lower referral rate cuts the overall cost of the screening program in half. An added benefit of a low false positive rate is fewer babies are lost to follow-up because there are fewer babies to follow. Consequently, the chance of losing a baby with hearing loss is less, which means the main goal of our screening program, to identify and get babies with hearing loss to intervention, has a higher probability of success.

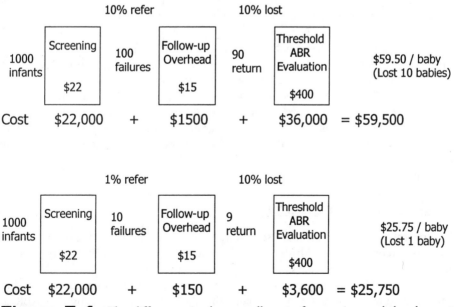

Figure 5-1   The difference in the overall cost of screening and the dropout rate caused by the referral rate of a screening program.

Third, the screening method should produce a consistent performance across operators with minimal training. Personnel are expensive to hire, train and retain. If a screening method requires little training for consistent performance, it will be less expensive. In addition, efficiency is improved if the screening instrument can function with as little interaction with the operator as possible. In other words, the instrument completes screenings while unattended.

Finally, a screening method should have a clear outcome, either the baby is ok or needs follow-up (translated to screening outcomes of pass and refer). Screening results that need to be interpreted are prone to error, inconsistency, and indecision. We have evaluated babies referred from other screening programs where the outcome of the screening was not clear to either the parents or the referring physician. The baby had either been screened so many times with conflicting results, or the results had been hedged in such a manner as to leave the parents and physician in a quandary. In addition, the need for interpretation of results greatly increases training costs.

The ALGO I Infant Hearing Screener was developed according to these criteria. We started using the ALGO, now referred to as automated ABR or AABR, in the nursery in 1984. It should be noted, however, that the term automated ABR is frequently used as an oblique way of referring to the ALGO hearing screeners manufactured by Natus Medical. Since the development of the ALGO, other *automated* ABR screening units have become available from other manufacturers. However, the automation incorporated into each unit is different and each instrument's screening performance needs to be assessed individually.

Since the development of commercial otoacoustic emissions (OAEs) equipment in the 1990s, we have evaluated the performance of OAEs for newborn hearing screening and found it is not equal to the performance standard we have achieved with the ALGO screeners. Primarily, we have found newborn hearing screening with OAEs to have a much higher false positive rate. Even with the most recent improvements in equipment, OAE referral rates are reported to be higher than those with the automated ABR, especially when performance is compared during the first 36 hours of life (Vohr, Carty, Moore, & Letourneau 1998; Jacobson & Jacobson 1994; Doyle, Fujikawa, Rogers, & Newman 1998). Although the number of false positives may be reduced by screening babies two or more times, this results in higher costs and also increases the probability of losing a baby with hearing loss in follow-up (Herrmann and Thornton, 1996). In addition, there may be a higher false negative rate with the OAE method (Vohr et al., 1998) than with the ABR as implemented in the ALGO screeners.

TEST PROTOCOL

The protocol used in our MGH screening protocol is shown in Figure 5–2. Each baby is screened once with the possible outcomes of pass in both ears, pass in one ear, or refer in both ears.

Babies who do not pass the screening in either ear (bilateral refers) are scheduled immediately for a complete threshold evaluation using the ABR at MEEI. Babies who pass in one or both ears are cleared for potential delays in speech and language development with the caution to retest if concerns arise

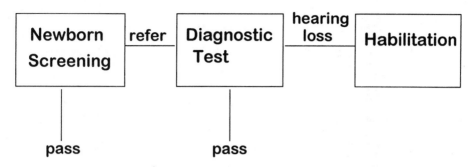

Figure 5-2 The protocol used in the newborn hearing screening program at the Massachusetts General Hospital Mother and Child Center and Neonatal Intensive Care nurseries.

later in development. The decision to follow only the bilateral refers is fairly unique and has been used since the inception of the program. It is based upon the logic that there is no intervention for unilateral hearing loss in the newborn period, and that unilateral hearing loss is not associated with delays in speech and language development. By concentrating our resources on following those babies at significant risk for speech and language delays, we decrease the number of babies to follow and, correspondingly, increase the probability of getting babies with hearing loss to intervention. Dropout in follow-up is also lessened by keeping the time between the screening and the diagnostic test as short as possible. We prefer to complete the evaluation before discharge, but if that is not possible we schedule the diagnostic evaluation within one week of discharge. The success of this strategy is shown by our screening statistics (Table 5–1). No babies failing the screening in both ears were lost to follow-up in 1998.

The steps used in implementing the protocol are kept simple and integrated with the Audiology Department's data systems. Each morning the nursery unit clerks provide the daily census of babies to the Audiology office, and each new baby is entered into a departmental database. A list of babies needing screening is generated for each nursery . The Level 3 screening list is adjusted in consultation with the NICU nurse manager regarding which babies are medically stable. We do not wait until NICU babies are near discharge for screening since we have found that once medically stable, screening results on NICU babies rarely change (Herrmann, Betero, Thornton, & Eavey, 1992). This strategy has reduced our missed screening rate in the NICU.

The medical record forms for documenting the screening are printed with the baby's demographics, eliminating the need for hand-labeling forms in the nursery. Screening lists and forms are placed in the Audiology patient cue for screening at 1:30 p.m., the time determined by the nursery and Audiology as the best routine time to screen. The first audiologist available at 1:30 p.m. takes responsibility for the screening. If there are a large number of babies in a day, two audiologists and up to four screeners (ALGO 1, 2 and 2e models) may be used. If a baby needs to be screened before 1:30 p.m., the nursery alerts Audiology and the screening times are adjusted as needed.

TABLE 5-1 Summary statistics for MGH Level 1 screening in 1998.

Month	Total Babies	Bilateral Pass	Unilateral Pass	Bilateral Refer	Babies Missed	Waived Babies	Follow-up Hearing Loss	Follow-up Normal	Lost to Follow-up
JAN	161	147	14	0	0	0	0	0	0
FEB	170	153	13	1	1	2	0	1	0
MAR	181	173	7	0	1	0	0	0	0
APR	172	163	7	2	0	0	1	1	0
MAY	177	172	5	0	0	0	0	0	0
JUN	167	155	12	0	0	0	0	0	0
JUL	198	187	10	0	0	1	0	0	0
AUG	230	215	14	1	0	0	0	1	0
SEP	170	158	12	0	0	0	0	0	0
OCT	201	192	9	0	0	0	0	0	0
NOV	206	191	12	1	2	0	1	0	0
DEC	197	185	10	0	2	0	0	0	0
TOTAL	2230	2091	125	5	6	3	2	3	0
(% of Total)		93.77%	5.61%	0.22%	0.27%	0.13%	0.09%	0.13%	0.00%

Babies in the Level 2 and Level 3 nurseries are tested at bedside. The nurse assigned to a Level 1 baby brings the infant to the Level 1 nursery. Several babies are brought at once, since the ALGO can screen accurately without input from the audiologist. The audiologist can then work efficiently by either prepping a baby or finishing the paperwork on another baby while a third baby is being screened. Experience has shown us that one audiologist can efficiently operate two screening instruments.

Results of each screening are marked on the form for the baby's medical record (Figure 5–3) and written on the daily screening list.

The medical record form is left in the baby's bassinet for the nurse to put into the MGH medical record and recorded into the MGH nursery systems. This form is sent with the other MGH records at discharge to the baby's pediatrician. A parent handout is also put in the bassinet for the parents of all babies passing the screening, explaining the screening and the results for that baby. Bilateral referral results are explained to the parents verbally with a parent handout used for reinforcement. The follow-up testing is scheduled and the primary physician is called.

Parents can decline the screening by signing the waiver at the bottom of the screening medical record form (Figure 5–3). Letters are sent to the primary physician and the parents of babies who are mistakenly discharged before being screened. The letter explains the situation and offers a screening in the Audiology Department.

Once all screenings are complete, the results are entered into the departmental database by our secretarial staff, and the billing information is exported for inclusion with the rest of the Audiology billing, which is uploaded to the MEEI Fiscal Department for billing to MGH. Each month, a screening report is generated that lists the number of babies tested, the number passing both ears, the number passing one ear, and the number referring in both ears (Table 5–1). The number of missed babies and the number of screens waived are also included, along with the follow-up statistics for bilateral referrals. Regular reporting of screening statistics helps monitor the quality of the screenings and follow-up, and helps to identify when problems may be present. It also helps to clear up misperceptions that sometimes arise among MEEI or MGH staff. For instance, when several babies require referral in close succession, it is easy to suspect that the screening is at fault. After ruling out any problems in the screening procedures, confidence in the screening can be maintained by showing that the number of referrals is still within the expected frequency.

COSTS/CHARGES

There are two types of costs in newborn hearing screening: the direct cost of doing the screening and the indirect costs of following screening referrals to diagnosis and, if necessary, intervention. The charge for the screening reflects the cost of personnel, supplies, equipment maintenance, and facility overhead. The personnel time includes time for doing the screening, for administration and supervision of the program, and for record keeping, including secretarial services. Of course, it is important to realize that full-time employee (FTE) cost for the personnel time needed must account for the indirect personnel costs related to time spent on vacation, sick leave, training, recruit-

AUDIOLOGIC EVALUATION

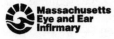
Massachusetts Eye and Ear Infirmary

	Boston	Stoneham
Audiology Clinic	573-3266	279-0864
Hearing Aid Center	573-4047	279-0943
AER Lab	573-3286	
FAX	573-3023	573-5644

Date:

Unit #:

Name:

Address:

D.O.B.:

Tested by:

MEEI - INFANT HEARING SCREENING PROGRAM

All babies born at Massachusetts General Hospital have a hearing screening before discharge as part of the routine care. The screening is done using Auditory Evoked Response with a click stimulus presented at 35 dB HL. An outcome of "Pass" in one or both ears indicates that the baby's hearing is adequate for speech and language development. An outcome of "Refer" indicates that further testing will be necessary in order to determine hearing sensitivity. Immediate follow-up will be required only in the case of a "Refer" in both ears because this is the only condition in which speech and language development is at risk.

OUTCOME

RIGHT EAR	Pass	Refer	Could not test

LEFT EAR	Pass	Refer	Could not test

RECOMMENDATIONS

____ Failed both ears. Immediate audiologic evaluation necessary.
Appointment will be scheduled by the Audiology Department, MEEI.

____ Passed one ear. No follow-up necessary for early speech and language development.
Retest on indications of hearing loss or delayed speech and language development.

____ Passed both ears. No immediate follow-up is needed.

FORM ID AU 4 '92

WAIVER

I have read and understood the description above.

I, _____ request that the newborn hearing screening not be done on my baby prior to discharge. I understand that early detection of hearing problems is important for the language development of my baby. I release the Massachusetts General Hospital and my physicians of any liability by requesting such and accept the responsibility for choosing not to have the screening done.

_____
Parent or Guardian

Figure 5-3 The medical record form used to report the result of newborn hearing screening. Documentation of a declined screening is made on the bottom of the form.

ment, etc., in addition to the amount of time directly spent in screening activities. We have also integrated institutional overhead costs (space, administration, utilities, capital depreciation, maintenance, purchasing, etc.) into our cost basis.

We calculate the personnel time for screening by using an estimated average of babies screened per hour. This includes equipment preparation, travel time to and from the nursery, set-up, documentation, and restocking consumables. A conservative estimate is approximately 3 babies per hour, which should not be confused with the screening test times. With the ALGO screener, our median test time per baby is 5 minutes; however, test times do not account for set-up, documentation, restocking, and travel time all of which must be included when estimating personnel time.

The cost of following screening referrals includes the cost of scheduling, confirming appointments, the diagnostic testing, and counseling visits afterwards. The fully loaded costs for these activities are the same as for any audiology patient and are incorporated into the regular charges for these tests and consultations. However, since the goal of our screening program is to identify babies with disabling hearing loss and to get those infants to intervention, there is an administrative cost to the program of following screening referrals. We try to minimize these costs by reducing the steps needed to get screening referrals to follow-up. Instead of letters and phone calls for babies needing a follow-up test, we schedule the follow-up appointment at the time of the screening. Preferably, the follow-up diagnostic test is scheduled within a week of the screening. The confirmation is then managed by our general procedures for AER threshold evaluations. The greater the number of referrals, the greater the administrative cost to the program, and the greater the overall cost to society for follow-up testing. Limiting the number of referrals through optimized methods and rational protocol decisions minimizes the cost.

COMMUNICATING WITH FAMILIES

Newborn hearing screening is part of the standard nursery routine at MGH, and, except in cases where follow-up is needed, communication occurs through the routine nursery channels, primarily the baby's nurse and the primary physician. Each family is given a brief description of the screening and its purpose in the prenatal packet. A baby's screening result is recorded for the family on a handout that explains what that result means (Figures 5–4A–D).

The handout for the unilateral passes includes answers to common questions about a unilateral pass result. Each handout also gives the telephone number of the Audiology Department at the Infirmary to provide answers for further questions. In addition, nurses are encouraged to call an audiologist to talk to any family with questions that he/she cannot answer. As described earlier, handouts for babies who pass in one or both ears are placed in the bassinet after the screening, and the nurse for each baby gives the result of the screening to the mother. The handouts for babies with refer results for both ears are given to the mother by the audiologist, who also verbally gives the results, answers any questions, and schedules the follow-up appointment.

FOLLOW-UP/FOLLOW-THROUGH

The screening program at MGH is designed to either complete or to have scheduled the first follow-up appointment, the threshold ABR evaluation, prior to hospital discharge. This minimizes the cost of follow-up by reducing the number of contact hours in scheduling, confirming, and tracking babies after discharge, as well as reducing the number of babies lost to follow-up.

Follow-up testing includes measurement of threshold sensitivity using the AER and, if needed, tympanometry and otoacoustic emissions. If the baby has normal hearing on follow-up, then the family can be confidently told that the hearing is fine and no further follow-up is needed. If the baby has a hearing loss, appropriate recommendations are made to the primary physician regarding otolaryngologic referral, and referral is made for audiologic management, which includes decisions regarding hearing aids and early intervention programs. Most often we follow these children immediately in Audiology through our Hearing Aid Center and Auditory Rehabilitation Center. This continuity of care reduces the dropout rate and, in many cases, our initial intervention serves as a transition to long-term care in other facilities. In some cases, the initial referrals are made to other audiologists and intervention programs.

Massachusetts General Hospital
MOTHER-CHILD UNIT
Newborn Hearing Screening

During your stay in the Mother-Child Unit at the Massachusetts General Hospital, your baby's hearing will be screened. The screening is done because hearing is important to your baby's growth and learning. Finding and acting on hearing difficulties early in life can help prevent many of the learning problems caused by hearing loss. The screening test is simple and safe. It measures your baby's brain waves in response to soft sounds presented to your baby through specially-designed earphones. The brain waves are picked up by sensors placed on your baby's head. The screening will determine if there is a need for a more extensive hearing test.

Although the screening usually takes about 15 minutes, it can last longer if your baby does not rest quietly. Your nurse will bring your baby to the nursery for the screening. In the nursery, an audiologist from the Massachusetts Eye and Ear Infirmary will screen your baby. The results of the screening will be given to you after the screening is completed and will be documented in your baby's medical record. If your baby needs any further testing after the screening, an audiologist will come and discuss that with you. If you have any questions about the hearing screening, feel free to ask your nurse to have the audiologist to come and discuss it with you. You can also call the Audiology Department at the Massachusetts Eye and Ear Infirmary (617-573-3266) and ask for an audiologist.

Figure 5-4A-D Handouts used to communicate screening results to families. Handout A is used in the prenatal packet. Handout B is used for a bilateral pass result. Handout C is used for a unilateral pass result. Handout D is used for a bilateral referral result, and is given by the audiologist with verbal reporting of the results and scheduling of a follow-up appointment.

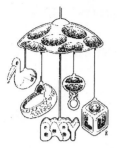

MASSACHUSETTS GENERAL HOSPITAL
MOTHER AND CHILD CENTER
NEWBORN HEARING SCREENING

To the parents of baby_____

It is a Massachusetts state law that all newborn babies be checked for hearing loss because good hearing is needed for a child to learn to talk.

Your baby passed the hearing test for both ears. This means that your baby's hearing should be adequate for normal speech and language development.

Children can develop hearing problems when they are older, so if you ever suspect that your child isn't hearing well, talk to your child's physician. If there is a family history of hearing loss, your child's hearing should be tested periodically.

If you have any questions about your baby's hearing screening, please call us, the Audiology Department at the **Massachusetts Eye and Ear Infirmary** (617-573-3266), and ask to speak to an audiologist.

Figure 5-4B

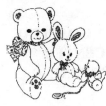

MASSACHUSETTS GENERAL HOSPITAL
MOTHER AND CHILD CENTER
NEWBORN HEARING SCREENING

To the parents of Baby_____

Your baby passed a hearing screening in the _____ ear only. Many parents have questions about their baby passing a screening in only one ear. The following are answers to some common questions.

Why was my baby's hearing tested?
Massachusetts state law requires infant hearing be tested because the only way to be sure that a baby hears well enough to learn to talk is to test each baby right after birth. This way any problems with hearing can be found early and many problems prevented. One normally-hearing ear is enough to learn to talk, so for learning purposes, your baby does not need any further testing now. Even if there was a problem with the ear that did not pass the screening, we would not do anything now.

Does this mean that my baby should be tested again right away?
Since one ear passed the hearing screening, we recommend that your baby be retested if you have concerns about speech and language development as your baby grows. Your baby's primary physician may have reasons to test your baby sooner, and you should discuss this issue with him or her. Of course, if at any time you suspect that your baby is not hearing well, talk to your baby's physician and have your baby's hearing tested right away.

How can I have my baby's hearing retested?
You can have your baby retested at the Audiology Department of the **Massachusetts Eye and Ear Infirmary** by calling to schedule a hearing test at 617-573-3266. Since many insurance plans restrict their coverage of health services to certain providers, we recommend that you talk to your baby's primary physician and check your insurance before scheduling a hearing test.

If you have further questions, you can ask your nurse to have an audiologist come and talk to you or you can call the Audiology Department at **Massachusetts Eye and Ear Infirmary** at 617-573-3266 and ask to speak to an audiologist.

Figure 5-4C

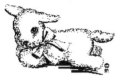

MASSACHUSETTS GENERAL HOSPITAL
MOTHER AND CHILD CENTER
NEWBORN HEARING SCREENING

To the parents of Baby _____

It is a Massachusetts state law that all newborn babies be checked for hearing loss because good hearing is needed for a child to learn to talk.

Your baby did not pass a hearing screening for either ear. This means that further testing is needed to see if there is a problem with your baby's hearing. This should be done within the next two weeks and most likely will be done before you leave the hospital or as you leave the hospital. An audiologist will talk to you today about your baby's hearing screening and make an appointment for the second test. It is important to keep this appointment because early detection can prevent many of the problems caused by hearing difficulties. If you have any questions, you may call the Audiology department at **Massachusetts Eye and Ear Infirmary** at 617-573-3266.

Figure 5–4D

CASE EXAMPLE 1: PASS

Baby A was born with no complications and admitted to the Level 1 nursery. She was screened the next day and passed in both ears. The screening result was recorded in her medical record using the standard form, which also was sent to the pediatrician upon her discharge (Figure 5–5). Her mother was given the handout explaining the results of the screening. She was discharged with the normal precautions for identification and treatment of later-onset hearing loss.

AUDIOLOGIC EVALUATION

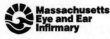 **Massachusetts Eye and Ear Infirmary**

	Boston	Stoneham
Audiology Clinic	573-3266	279-0864
Hearing Aid Center	573-4047	279-0943
AER Lab	573-3286	
FAX	573-3023	573-5644

Date:

Unit #:

Name: **Baby A**

Address:

D.O.B.:

Tested by:

MEEI - INFANT HEARING SCREENING PROGRAM

All babies born at Massachusetts General Hospital have a hearing screening before discharge as part of the routine care. The screening is done using Auditory Evoked Response with a click stimulus presented at 35 dB HL. An outcome of "Pass" in one or both ears indicates that the baby's hearing is adequate for speech and language development. An outcome of "Refer" indicates that further testing will be necessary in order to determine hearing sensitivity. Immediate follow-up will be required only in the case of a "Refer" in both ears because this is the only condition in which speech and language development is at risk.

OUTCOME

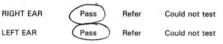

RIGHT EAR   Pass   Refer   Could not test

LEFT EAR   Pass   Refer   Could not test

RECOMMENDATIONS

____ Failed both ears. Immediate audiologic evaluation necessary.
Appointment will be scheduled by the Audiology Department, MEEI.

____ Passed one ear. No follow-up necessary for early speech and language development.
Retest on indications of hearing loss or delayed speech and language development.

_X_ Passed both ears. No immediate follow-up is needed.

WAIVER

I have read and understood the description above.

I, _____ request that the newborn hearing screening not be done on my baby prior to discharge. I understand that early detection of hearing problems is important for the language development of my baby. I release the Massachusetts General Hospital and my physicians of any liability by requesting such and accept the responsibility for choosing not to have the screening done.

_____
Parent or Guardian

FORM ID AU 4 '92

AUDIOLOGY

Figure 5-5 Medical record form for Case 1, a baby with a bilateral pass result.

CASE EXAMPLE 2: REFER

Baby B was admitted to the NICU immediately after birth. She was screened for hearing loss on day 4 of life and did not pass in either ear. The screening result was recorded using the standard form for her medical record (Figure 5–6A) and an appointment was made for a threshold auditory-evoked response evaluation the next day. The result of that evaluation (Figure 5–6B) indicated a moderate-to-severe sensorineural hearing loss in both ears.

Her parents were counseled and scheduled to return for additional rehabilitation counseling the following week. Concurrently, the patient was referred to a pediatric otolaryngologist on staff. The infant was enrolled in our Auditory Rehabilitation program for speech and language intervention. She was also enrolled in our Pediatric Amplification Loaner (PAL) program and was fit at 20 days of age with a body-style hearing aid, with the receiver coupled to tubing and placed behind the pinna. Initial wearing times were targeted for her non-sleeping hours. We frequently use a body-style hearing aid for infants to reduce the problems with earmold fitting and feedback. When appropriate for the hearing loss, the style of the hearing aid is changed when the child grows and the pinna can better accommodate a behind-the-ear style of amplification, without feedback and frequent earmold changes. Baby B is showing good responsiveness to amplification. Her parents are learning to be skilled facilitators of speech and language.

AUDIOLOGIC EVALUATION

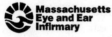

Massachusetts Eye and Ear Infirmary

	Boston	Stoneham
Audiology Clinic	573-3266	279-0864
Hearing Aid Center	573-4047	279-0943
AER Lab	573-3286	
FAX	573-3023	573-5644

Date:

Unit #:

Name: **Baby B**

Address:

D.O.B.:

Tested by:

MEEI - INFANT HEARING SCREENING PROGRAM

All babies born at Massachusetts General Hospital have a hearing screening before discharge as part of the routine care. The screening is done using Auditory Evoked Response with a click stimulus presented at 35 dB HL. An outcome of "Pass" in one or both ears indicates that the baby's hearing is adequate for speech and language development. An outcome of "Refer" indicates that further testing will be necessary in order to determine hearing sensitivity. Immediate follow-up will be required only in the case of a "Refer" in both ears because this is the only condition in which speech and language development is at risk.

OUTCOME

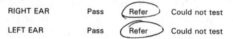

RIGHT EAR	Pass	(Refer)	Could not test
LEFT EAR	Pass	(Refer)	Could not test

RECOMMENDATIONS

X̲ Failed both ears. Immediate audiologic evaluation necessary. Appointment will be scheduled by the Audiology Department, MEEI.

___ Passed one ear. No follow-up necessary for early speech and language development. Retest on indications of hearing loss or delayed speech and language development.

___ Passed both ears. No immediate follow-up is needed.

WAIVER

I have read and understood the description above.

I, _____ request that the newborn hearing screening not be done on my baby prior to discharge. I understand that early detection of hearing problems is important for the language development of my baby. I release the Massachusetts General Hospital and my physicians of any liability by requesting such and accept the responsibility for choosing not to have the screening done.

_____
Parent or Guardian

FORM ID AU 4 '92

AUDIOLOGY

Figure 5-6A Medical record form for Case 2, a baby with a bilateral refer result.

AUDITORY EVOKED RESPONSE LABORATORY

DATE TESTED:	INTERPRETATION BY:
UNIT #:	
NAME: Baby B	
D.O.B.:	MEDICATIONS ORDERED BY: See medication order

EAR STIMULATED		AD	AD	AD		AS	AS	AS		BC	BC				
STIMULUS TYPE		B	B	C		B	B	B		B	C				
FREQUENCY (Hz)		1000	2000	– – –		1000	2000	4000		2000	– – –				
INTENSITY RANGE PROBED IN dB HL	LOW	80	70	75		55	70	80		30	45				
	HIGH	90	97	85		70	90	97		52	57				
LOWEST INTENSITY THAT RESPONSE WAS PRESENT		90	90	85		60	75	90		NR	50				

KEY:		ESTIMATED HEARING THRESHOLD SENSITIVITY									
AD=RIGHT EAR AS=LEFT EAR BC=BONE		FOR PURE TONES						FOR BEST FREQUENCY IN RANGE SHOWN			
		500	1000	2000	4000	8000		FREQ. RANGE	THRESH.	FREQ. RANGE	THRESH.
CONDUCTION C=CLICK	RIGHT EAR		85	90				500–8000	80		
S=SINE B=BURST	LEFT EAR		60	75	85						
HPC=HIGH–PASS CLICK	BINAURAL										
BPC=BAND–PASS CLICK	BONE COND. (FOREHEAD)			NR				500–8000	45		
*=CONTRALATERAL MASKING USED											

Sleep was induced with chloral hydrate taken orally.

INTERPRETATIONS:
Results indicate moderate to severe hearing loss in the left ear and a severe hearing loss in the right ear. This hearing loss is handicapping for speech and language development. Amplification is recommended.

Patient will be followed otologically and audiologically at the Massachusetts Eye and Ear Infirmary.

Figure 5-6B Report of threshold auditory-evoked response evaluation for Case 2, a baby with bilateral refer result.

REFERENCES

Doyle, K., Fujikawa, S., Rogers, P., & Newman, E. (1998). Comparison of newborn hearing screening by transient otoacoustic emissions and auditory brainstem response using ALGO-2. *International Journal of Pediatric Otorhinolaryngology, 43*, 207–11.

Herrmann, B., & Thornton, A. (1996). Audiologic follow-up after failure of an infant hearing screening. *Current Opinion in Otolaryngology and Head and Neck Surgery, 4*, 367–370.

Herrmann, B., Betero, M., Thornton, A., & Eavey, R. (1992). Monitoring NICU infants by multiple ABR automated screenings. *ASHA (a), 34,* 209.

Herrmann, B., Thornton, A., & Joseph, J. (1995). Automated infant hearing screening using the ABR: Development and validation. *American Journal of Audiology, 4*, 6–14.

Jacobson J., & Jacobson, C. (1994). The effects of noise in transient EOAE newborn hearing screening. *International Journal of Pediatric Otorhinolaryngology, 29*, 235–248.

Sprague, B., & Thornton, A. (1979). Simplified infant hearing screening using middle-component auditory-evoked responses. *ASHA (a), 21,* 735.

Thornton, A. (1978). Improved detection of auditory evoked potentials. *ASHA (a), 20,* 765.

Thornton, A., & Obenour, J. (1981). Auditory response detection and apparatus. *United States Patent #4.275.744,* 1981. Reviewed in *Journal of Acoustics Society of America, 10,* 1814.

Vohr, B., Carty, L., Moore, P., & Letourneau, K. (1998). The Rhode Island Hearing Assessment Program: Experience with statewide hearing screening (1993–1996). *Journal of Pediatrics,* Sept. 353–357.

The Sounds of Texas: Newborn Hearing Screening Using Otoacoustic Emissions

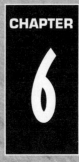

CHAPTER

6

Terese Finitzo, Ph.D.
Wendy Crumley, M.S.

INTRODUCTION

Universal newborn hearing screening (UNHS) is one step in the process of Early Hearing Detection and Intervention (EHDI). UNHS is the hospital-based component where screening for hearing should occur. EHDI encompasses the entire process from detection in the nursery to connection to services; audiologic, medical, developmental, and educational. This chapter describes two model UNHS programs using otoacoustic emissions, one utilizing distortion product otoacoustic emissions (DPOAE) and another utilizing transient evoked otoacoustic emissions (TEOAE). The hospitals are both in the state of Texas with annual births of 800 to 1,800. They have Level 1 and Level 2 nurseries with no Neonatal Intensive Care Unit (NICU). Sick and premature infants are transferred to the nearest affiliated hospital or to the children's hospital.

The primary goal of these model hospital-based programs is simple: to offer hearing screening to 100% of newborns during their birth admission, and to provide a mechanism to screen any infant missed at birth before they are one month of age. The equally critical second goal is to assure that there is a robust link between the birth admission screening program and the follow-up diagnostic and intervention service. Experience has taught us that this second goal is the one most difficult to achieve. Yet without it, there is no reason to screen for hearing during the birth admission.

In order to achieve these goals in any hospital program, we learned early of the need for effective information management. The issue of information management has been foremost since early 1994 when our team of audiologists began to assume management responsibility for multiple hospital screening programs. Our audiologic team worked with Dr. Kenneth Pool, a neurologist and programmer, to develop a tool that met our needs as audiologists. Information management should answer four questions. 1) What is the status of an individual infant? 2) Which babies need rescreening, audiologic evaluation, and intervention? 3) How are the hospital's individual screeners performing? 4) How is the overall program performing? That tool is now a commercial product, the OZ Corporation's Screening and Information Management Solution (OZ SIMS©, 1995–1999), and is being used in all our programs. We will not institute a program without effective information management as our professional credibility and liability are at stake.

While a UNHS program may have a medical director, the audiologist functions as the program manager or supervisor responsible for all aspects of screening including training, reporting, and documentation. Each of the model programs described here has a pediatrician as medical director and an audiologist who is a member of our project team. The medical director leaves all management decisions to the audiologist who informs him/her of any issues that affect infants and their families, medical colleagues, or program quality.

UNHS is a new program in most hospitals, including our model programs and as such, we had the opportunity to create and develop them from the ground up. Introducing any new program at a time when hospitals are overwhelmed with demands necessitates careful consideration of technical and personnel issues. Thus, prior to implementing the UNHS programs, an audiologist conducted environmental assessments of the hospitals' preparedness to introduce this new service. The environmental assessment is a partnership effort with the medical and nursery staff and administrative personnel in the hospital to address the following issues:

1. Target hearing loss including expected incidence
2. Target population
3. Instrumentation and technology decisions
4. Screening environment
5. Personnel
6. Day-to-day screening protocols
7. Case examples
8. Communication and documentation
9. Tracking and follow-up
10. Quality indicators and outcome measurements

Once the environmental assessment is complete, a document can be generated, providing a road map for all involved. Such a map can take the form of policy and procedures or a guideline for the program. We have found the environmental assessment to be a mechanism to achieve consensus among staff with differing levels of knowledge. Moreover, it can be beneficial when questions of accountability and responsibility arise. An administrator is unlikely to discontinue a program that identifies 3 infants in 1,000 to 1,500 screened if it is understood that this is the expected outcome. When outcomes are established in advance, program performance is readily evaluated.

TARGET HEARING LOSS

The target hearing loss is one that can interfere with the normal development of communication skills. It is a permanent, unilateral, or bilateral hearing loss of approximately 30 to 40 dB HL or greater in the speech frequencies. The targeted hearing loss is either sensory or conductive in nature. The incidence of this degree of loss is between 2 and 3 per 1,000 newborns screened. In our experience 75% of the losses are bilateral and 25% are unilateral.

A decision must be made regarding whether conductive hearing loss caused by otitis media is included in the target hearing loss. While transient conductive hearing loss from otitis media is important, we run the risk of derailing programs if our stated goal includes identifying all infants with conductive hearing losses. The sheer number of infants who need to be followed may increase costs to the point that administrators, who currently receive little financial remuneration for the program, will consider eliminating the program. The added controversy about otitis media management among pediatricians must also be considered. We want, indeed, we *need* their support in this effort. A given program may elect to follow and manage this group of infants if sufficient financial and pediatric support are available.

A decision must also be made regarding whether auditory neuropathy is included in the target hearing loss. Auditory neuropathy is characterized clinically by absent or abnormal auditory brainstem responses in the presence of normal TEOAEs or DPOAEs. Many of the infants who have been identified with this disorder are NICU graduates with hyperbilirubinemia resulting in a transfusion. The disorder is on a continuum with some infants showing recovery, others demonstrating minimal communication sequelae, and some with severe communication disorders but varying responses to amplification and therapy. At this time, auditory neuropathy is not well characterized. In the model programs described here, without a NICU, the decision to use OAEs is also a decision not to include auditory neuropathy in the target hearing loss; however, many of our larger nurseries, with several thousand annual births and a NICU, do use screening or diagnostic ABR in the NICU, in an effort to identify these infants as needing further care.

TARGET POPULATION

Since an estimated 40% to 50% of infants have no known risk factors for hearing loss, the target population is *all* newborns. All newborns are to be screened during their birth admission. If a newborn is discharged early and screening does not occur, hospitals need to have a mechanism for identifying these newborns and offering a screening within one month post-discharge.

Despite the absence of a NICU in the programs described here, it should be noted that NICU graduates might fall outside the target definition for several reasons. First, an infant's prematurity or medical condition may prohibit effective screening prior to a chronological age of one month. A baby with a gestational age of 29 to 34 weeks will have a higher incidence of transient auditory abnormalities, including fluid in the middle ear and/or brainstem pathway dysfunction. Second, a NICU graduate may actually be a transfer from another hospital's nursery. Even if screened before transfer, the infant's condition will usually warrant a second screen or assessment before discharge from the NICU. Some infants are transferred back to their original nursery, but this may be another source of disconnection for a family. Hence, it may be necessary to have a mechanism in place that assures all NICU infants are screened before discharge from that NICU. If an infant is to be transferred back to the original nursery, documentation and communication to the medical and nursery staff should accompany the transfer. In the model hospitals described here, since neither has a NICU, both send infants to an affiliated hospital or children's hospital's NICU. Thus, it was necessary to document and track these babies in the referral process.

The target population also includes all infants who need ongoing medical surveillance for delayed onset or progressive hearing loss. While tracking these infants to monitor their hearing status may not be the responsibility of the birthing hospital, it is the hospital's responsibility to document infants with known risk indicators for progressive or incident-based hearing loss so that they may be tracked. In our experience to date, this usually happens for the NICU infants whose medical conditions are better recognized. But it must happen for all infants, as hereditary involvement and cytomegalovirus are two conditions that may produce progressive or delayed onset losses. In many cases, the information is simply not known and in others it has not been feasible because of the time constraints involved in requiring screening staff to interview parents regarding familial histories.

INSTRUMENTATION AND TECHNOLOGY DECISIONS

A hospital can implement a UNHS program successfully with either otoacoustic emissions or auditory brainstem responses. Other factors, usually personnel issues, cause a program to succeed or fail, *not* technology. That said, our statewide program currently has thirty-five active hospitals. The technology mix includes: four using TEOAE and screening ABR (SABR), fourteen using DPOAE and SABR, twelve using DPOAE only, two using TEOAE only, and two using SABR only. Technology is changing rapidly and this description is not an endorsement of any specific technology. There are clear pros and cons to each technology decision. For this chapter, two model otoacoustic emissions programs are described, one using DPOAE only and one using TEOAE only.

Otoacoustic Emissions

More and more manufacturers of otoacoustic emissions have automated interpretation algorithms that can be used in nursery testing. Some manufacturers allow the user to establish the interpretive criteria. Other manufacturers provide pre-established pass/refer criteria. Every automated interpretation, regardless of technology, should be accompanied by a clear scientific rationale that is either statistically based or experientially derived. Either way, it is essential to understand the protocols and their underlying assumptions. It must be recognized that every protocol decision, including the number of frequencies sampled, number of samples in the averaging process, frequency ratio, intensity level, minimum dB amplitude, signal-to-noise ratio, and number of exams, will affect the sensitivity and specificity. If the automated algorithm is based on statistics and signal detection theory, these rates can be estimated. If the pass/refer criteria are empirically based, then estimating sensitivity and specificity becomes difficult to measure and control.

DPOAE Technical Considerations

Once the decision to use DPOAE as the screening technology has been made, the audiologist must determine the collection parameters, including what constitutes a pass. We use the OZ SIMS© interpretive algorithm. DPOAEs can be recorded reliably in neonates in response to stimuli above 1000 Hz. The current protocol in use in our model program is to vary the higher frequency tone (F2) from 4800 Hz to 2400 Hz and the F1 tone from 4000 to 2000 Hz. The F2/F1 ratio of 1.22 typically results in the greatest amplitude distortion product (DP), which is the emission returning from the cochlea to the microphone (see Chapters 1 and 2). We sample five stimuli pairs for each ear, and require that 4 of 5 meet the pass criteria for an ear to pass the screen. The DP is measured at a mathematically defined location (0.8 of F1), based upon the cubic difference formula, 2F1–F2. This formula is generally the most prominent cubic difference tone. The surrounding noise floor is also measured and incorporated into the pass/refer criteria. The OZ SIMS© algorithm examines multiple points on either side of the DP, producing a more stable estimate of noise than if just one or two points are measured. The difference in amplitude between the surrounding noise and the DP is the signal-to-noise ratio (SNR). The intensity of the high frequency is 65 dB (L1) and 55 dB (L2) for the lower of the two frequencies. Generally, intensities above 75 dB are not recommended as the possibility of an acoustic DP derived solely from the ear canal increases. An alternative to a statistical algorithm is a preset empirical algorithm with an absolute minimum dB amplitude or minimum signal-to-noise ratio to constitute a pass for a frequency, and a preset number of frequencies to pass the hearing screening in that ear.

For DPOAE, the OZ SIMS© algorithm measures the probability that a response is present with sensitivity calculated to be at least 99.99%. The algorithm accounts for number of frequencies (5 for DPOAE); number required to pass (4 for DPOAE); number of allowable exams (a maximum of 8 total for two ears prior to referral for diagnostic audiological evaluation); and the follow-up protocol (we follow and rescreen unilateral fails). A limited number of multiple exams are allowed because the infant may fail a screening because of debris from the ear canal in the probe tip, or because of excessive noise from the environment or the infant. The defaults produce an average exam time of 35 to 45 seconds per trial. The beauty of the algorithm is that an audiologist can exercise professional judgment and modify any of these parameters while maintaining the preset sensitivity. It is the specificity that varies with the above protocol decisions.

TEOAE Technical Considerations

Once the decision to use TEOAE as the screening technology has been made, the audiologist must determine the collection parameters, including what constitutes a pass. After placement of a probe in the infant's ear canal, 80 microsecond electric pulses are applied to the transducer at a 78 to 83 dB peak equivalent sound pressure level (SPL). Responses are recorded for sets of four stimuli; three in phase and one out of phase, with the other three and at an intensity level three times that of the other three. This presentation mode produces an average response that reduces stimulus artifact and the linear components of the ear's response to the transient stimulus. The response from one set of stimuli is stored in buffer "A," the second in "B," with sampling continuing for a predetermined number of minimum sweeps.

The following steps describe the interface with OZ SIMS©, which exemplifies the pass criteria in our model TEOAE program. First, technical adequacy of the screening trial is determined. Stimulus intensity cannot exceed 85 dB SPL during screening. Thus, the infant cannot pass the screen inadvertently because of an unrecognized excessive stimulus level. A minimum of 70 quiet sweeps must be collected. If these two criteria are not met, the trial is considered technically inadequate for evaluation.

If a trial is technically adequate, three criteria are necessary for an infant to pass the hearing screen. First, whole wave reproducibility, or the value of the cross-correlation between buffers A and B, has to be at least 50%. Second, a minimum signal-to-noise ratio of 6 dB at 4000 Hz is required. The signal-to-noise ratio is computed as the difference between the fast Fourier transform components common to both A and B buffers (the true emission) and those components not present in both buffers (noise). Third, two of three additional signal-to-noise ratios must be met, a minimum of 6 dB at 2400 and 3200 Hz and 3 dB at 1600 Hz. If all three of these criteria are achieved, the trial is a pass and there is no further evaluating. If a trial does not meet the criteria for a pass, it is first examined for technical adequacy. If either stimulus intensity is 60 dB SPL or stimulus stability is <75%, the trial is classified as technically inadequate. If neither of these is present, the trial is considered a refer or fail. The average exam time with these relatively stringent pass criteria is 110 to 128 seconds per trial.

SCREENING ENVIRONMENT

There are often few alternatives to choose for the hearing screening environment. In some cases, all screening occurs in the nursery itself. When evaluating a site, examiners should stand in the space and "listen to" the area where screening is to occur. Is there a noisy ventilation system nearby? Is there likely to be electrical noise arising from nearby spaces? Is it a high traffic area? The model programs described here conduct screening in a quiet room off the main nursery. Sound level measurements during screening were taken prior to beginning the program. In our experience, however, sound level meter measurements are not necessary if the visual and auditory check of the space do not reveal problems.

PERSONNEL

Throughout our hospital programs, various personnel are employed to screen hearing: neonatal nurse practitioners, nurses, respiratory and EEG technicians, and unit assistants. We do not advocate the use of volunteers. If newborn hearing screening is to be a serious national effort, it cannot succeed with volunteers. In fact, many hospitals are prohibited from billing when volunteers are used. In larger hospitals there are often dedicated screening personnel. Smaller hospitals, including the model sites described here, have cross-trained staff to cover screening. We train only as many staff as are necessary to cover the nursery seven days per week. A typical program has four nursing staff available to screen infants. Too large a staff reduces the quality of the program, as none of the screeners develop the expertise needed, especially in hospitals with small birth rates and limited opportunities for staff to gain experience.

Following inservice for screening personnel, we monitor individual performance via OZ SIMS©. OZ SIMS©, as the "manager" of the data, keeps track of screener performance for key DPOAE and TEOAE collection parameters. This enables the supervising audiologist to monitor the performance of each screener. It also allows individual screening personnel to monitor their own performance. Of course, if a screener's statistics are not improving, the audiologist returns for focused re-education in the problem areas. With OAE testing, this re-education usually includes addressing probe fitting problems. Probe fitting problems can introduce too much noise in an exam and result in a high technical fail rate for a screener.

DAY-TO-DAY SCREENING PROTOCOLS

Once personnel decisions are made, screening staff are trained in the day-to-day screening protocols and the nursery manager is instructed on how to undertake simple program review. Figure 6–1 displays the hearing screening protocol followed in both programs. The audiologist functions as the program manager, assuming responsibility for tracking and follow-up. Basic training on the OZ SIMS© and DPOAE or TEOAE systems takes one to two days.

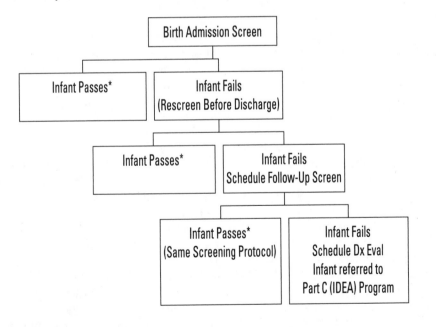

*Infants who have risk factors for delayed onset or progressive hearing loss will be reevaluated on a periodic basis.

Figure 6-1 Hearing screening protocol for otoacoustic emissions.

The screener is instructed to obtain the nursery intake list of newly admitted babies and enter the new patient information into the OZ SIMS© pending list. Newer systems may upload hospital records directly into OZ SIMS©. The basic demographics that need to be entered include the baby's last name, gender, permanent medical record number, and date of birth. Other demographics such as time of birth, gestational age, nursery level, and care location can be included. The baby's new medical home, that is, the primary care physician or Medicaid Clinic of record, can be selected from a standard Window® drop-down menu in OZ SIMS©. Much of the demographic information defaults to the most frequent entry, such as 38 to 40 weeks gestational age, which is the normal gestational age for infants. Most hospitals elect to enter parent contact information into OZ SIMS© only if the newborn fails the birth admission screen, is transferred to another hospital for NICU care, or has a known risk indicator for delayed-onset or progressive hearing loss.

Next, the screener is instructed on the OAE system. We strongly advise daily calibration of the OAE probe to ensure the infant is screened with a functioning probe. If a system is not calibrated within a predetermined intervening time, the system is automatically disabled until calibration is complete. In our experience, both the DPOAE and TEOAE systems have proven easy to learn. Probe placement in every OAE system requires practice to become a proficient screener. While the probes are relatively robust, they are the weak link in the system. Thus, we spend time teaching the screening staff how to care for and maintain the probe. An advantage of using OAEs over ABR is that the disposable supply cost for the probe tips is significantly less. Most hospitals elect to use a new tip for each infant rather than deal with sterilization issues. As mentioned above, test time is rapid.

If an infant passes the initial screen, hearing care is considered complete unless there are risk indicators. If an infant does not pass the initial screen, it is repeated before discharge, preferably several hours later. Hence, our protocol is a "Texas two-step" regardless of the technology mix. We also teach personnel not to rescreen an infant too often. If a baby fails an exam repeatedly (defined by our protocol), referral is needed. The interpretive algorithm in OZ SIMS© informs a screener if the exam is a pass, refer, or technically inadequate exam. A technically inadequate exam occurs when the environment or the baby is too noisy, the minimum number of sweeps were not collected, or the stimuli exceeded the recommended dB level. Therefore, screeners can improve their screening technique to improve the outcome. If the infant repeatedly does not pass, screening should be discontinued. We have all been indoctrinated about false positive outcomes, yet we forget that each exam is a new "roll of the dice." Over-screening will only increase the chance of a false negative outcome.

The daily protocol requires that a report for each newborn be generated from OZ SIMS©. As part of the basic program set-up, the audiologist customizes the report content for the new medical home (the primary care provider), the parent, and the hospital's medical record. As screeners in these two hospitals are also nurses or unit secretaries, the audiologist has carefully instructed them as to how the screening results should be conveyed to parents. Education focuses on the importance of follow-up and use of terminology appropriate for communication with families. Since many areas in our state have high transient populations, communicating results before discharge ensures that all families will be informed of screening results in a timely manner.

CASE EXAMPLES

DPOAE Pass

Figure 6–2A is the DP gram for the right ear of a newborn. Note that the Pass result indicates that the infant passed the birth admission screen in this ear at all five frequencies. Note the table with corresponding values in Figure 6–2B. The first column is the frequency of F1 with the corresponding L1 in column 2. Column 3 is the F2 frequency followed in column 4 by the actual intensity measured at the microphone for this test. The DP frequency (DP HZ) is shown next. Remember, it is 0.8 of F1. The absolute DP (DP dB) is next with the noise floor in column 7 and the noise variance in column 8. The signal-to-noise ratio is shown as DP net and the standard deviation of the signal-to-noise ratio is in the final column. For this newborn, the signal-to-noise ratio (dB net) are 25.20 dB at 2437 Hz (corresponding to F2), 27.10 dB at 2875 Hz, 27.70 dB at 3437 Hz, 24.80 dB at 4125 Hz, and 20.60 dB at 4875 Hz.

DPOAE Refer

Figures 6–3A and 6–3B are the DP gram and corresponding values in table form from OZ SIMS©, for an infant who did not pass the birth admission screen. Data show that the baby did not pass 4 out of 5 of the frequency sets used in analysis. The noise floor is not an issue with this infant as noise and standard deviation (SD) of the noise are relatively low. The signal-to-noise ratio (dB net) are 7.40 dB at 2437 Hz (corresponding to F2), 3.40 dB at 2875 Hz, −4.20 dB at 3437 Hz, −5.70 dB at 4125 Hz, and 1.70 dB at 4875 Hz. Only the single frequency signal-to-noise ratio (dB net) at 2437 Hz would be adequate; however, the exam in total is a Refer.

TEOAE Pass

Figure 6–4A is the TEOAE graph for the left ear of an infant. The top left hand corner of the graph is a visual display of the stimuli being presented into the infant's ear. The bottom left hand corner is the frequency response of the emission from the ear. The middle box represents the response from the infant's ear with the hatched area being the noise from the patient or the environment, and the solid area being the emission from the ear. The noise floor slopes from the left to the right because there is more noise present at lower frequencies. The box on the right hand side is another display of the amplitude of the emission plotted in dB gain without the noise floor. Clearly, a TEOAE response is present. Figure 6–4B is the tabular form with corresponding values. Note, this infant met the criteria of a minimum of 70 quiet sweeps, stimulus stability of 70% or greater, whole wave reproducibility of 50% or greater, and the stimulus was maintained between 78 and 80 dB SPL. Therefore, this infant passed the screening in the left ear.

TEOAE Refer

Figures 6–5A and 6–5B are the TEOAE graph and corresponding values in tabular form for an infant who did not pass the birth admission screen in the left ear. In the graph, a very minimal emission displayed by the amount of solid area above the noise floor (hatched area) is detected. However, the infant met the other criteria of a minimum of 70 quiet sweeps, stimulus stability of 70% or greater, and the stimulus did not exceed 85 dB SPL. Therefore, this infant did not pass the screening in the left ear.

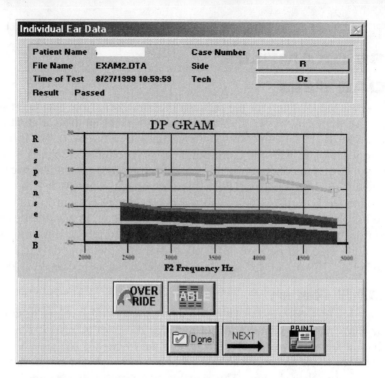

Figure 6-2 DP-gram (upper) and corresponding tabular data (lower) for an infant who passed the birth admission DPOAE screen in the right ear at all five frequencies.

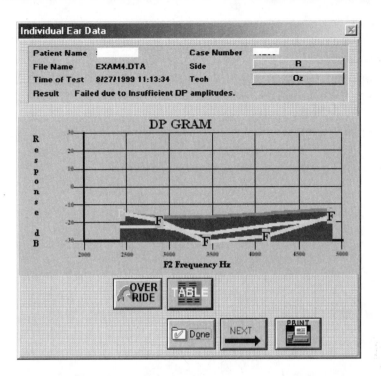

Figure 6-3 DP-gram (upper) and corresponding tabular data (lower) for an infant who did *not* pass the birth admission DPOAE screen at four of the five frequencies.

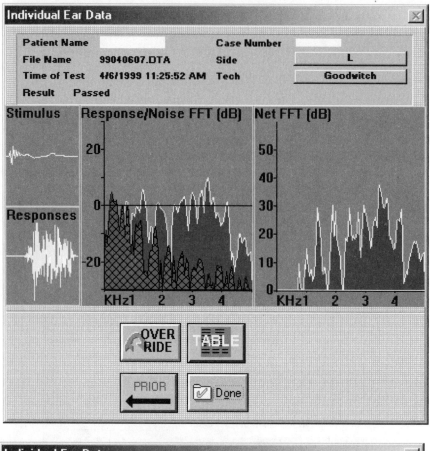

Figure 6-4 Graph of transient evoked otoacoustic emissions (upper) and corresponding tabular data (lower) for an infant who passed the birth admission TEOAE screen in the left ear.

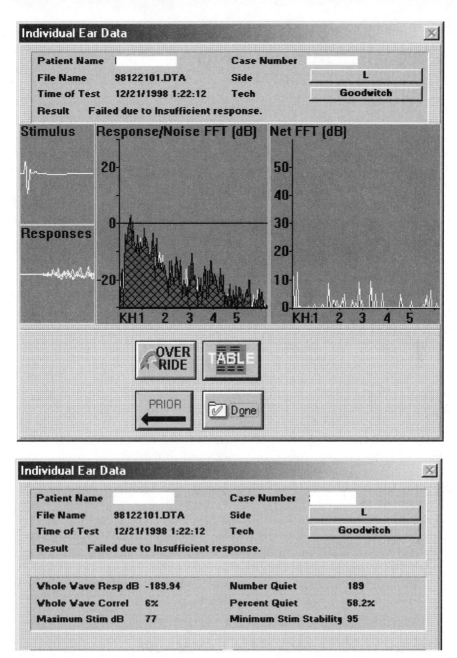

Figure 6-5 Graph of transient evoked otoacoustic emissions (upper) and corresponding tabular data (lower) for an infant who did not pass the birth admission TEOAE screen in the left ear.

COMMUNICATION AND DOCUMENTATION

Communication begins with information to parents provided at the prenatal education classes and/or through pre-registration packets. The audiologist provides the nurse educators with a set of overheads that summarizes key points on screening. This information must be delivered in a short time, since Lamaze/prenatal educators have much information to include in a limited number of classes. Parents also take home a brochure on communication milestones with their hearing screening results to review at their leisure. In hospitals with a high teen pregnancy rate, the high school nurse has also been given information on hearing screening.

Before program implementation, the audiologist makes a presentation to the medical staff. In addition, all medical staff receive a brochure in their office, informing them of the new service. Similarly, nursery personnel who are not screeners receive an in-service on early identification of hearing loss. Once nurses and physicians are aware of the advantages of the screening, they are almost always program advocates.

The OZ SIMS© system generates reports and confirms that the new medical home, parent, and medical record have been generated and are up to date, as well as whether new testing has been undertaken. In one instance, an infant did not pass his birth admission screening and the parent gave the wrong phone number and address to the hospital. The family canceled the first follow-up screening appointment. This family could not be reached via phone or mail because of incorrect information. The screener was able to document that the mother had canceled her first appointment and that efforts had been made to reach this family to schedule a follow-up appointment. The system automatically dates and time stamps each note and keeps track of the infant's need for follow-up. Thus, documentation of the hospital's effort was clear. When the baby finally returned to the primary care provider, the physician had a letter and report stating that the infant had not passed the birth admission hearing screening and was considered lost to follow-up. In this case, the infant had a severe bilateral hearing loss. Thanks to the physician's and hospital staff's diligent efforts, the infant was fitted with amplification at 6 months of age. Such documentation is critical for accurate program evaluation and for liability purposes.

TRACKING AND FOLLOW-UP

Effective information management facilitates tracking and follow-up. In the INFO "page" in OZ SIMS©, each baby's evaluation status is shown. Thus, the first issue on the status of a baby can be answered by reviewing this page. Is a baby's birth screen complete? Is follow-up pending? What is the date of follow-up?

The second issue is to know which babies need care of some kind. In OZ SIMS©, this is an advanced program manager capability. Sorting or filtering capabilities to identify infants who meet certain criteria are available. In this way, the audiologist in our model site is able to identify all babies each month who failed or did not receive a screening at birth, and who have not yet returned for follow-up.

In the programs described here, it is the hospital staff that provides follow-up re-screening, if needed, one to two weeks later for infants who did not pass the birth admission screen. However, it is ideal to have the audiologist available for follow-up care, as it is at this stage that parents need expert counseling on audiologic, medical, and developmental assessment and intervention. If the infant does not pass at this stage of screening, a transfer packet of all the baby's data is created in OZ SIMS© and shipped via modem to the audiologic referral site for continued management of the child.

QUALITY INDICATORS AND OUTCOME MEASUREMENTS

Quality indicators are used to monitor outcomes at each step in the EHDI process. Quality indicators reflect a result in relation to a stated target. We monitor quality using well-established practices of statistical process control to determine program consistency and stability. Recall that as part of the environmental assessment, programs come to a decision regarding the quality indicators they will monitor. The two hospitals described here chose:

- Percentage of infants screened during the birth admission.
- Percentage of infants screened before one month of age.
- Percentage of infants who do not pass the birth admission screen.
- Percentage of infants who return for follow-up testing (either follow-up screening or diagnostic audiological evaluation and medical evaluation).
- Percentage of infants who are referred for diagnostic audiological services.

The benchmarks we provide for the chosen indicators function as targets to evaluate the hospital's progress. They are:

- To screen 95% of all infants within one year (our experience is that programs can achieve and maintain this outcome even with birth admissions of 24 hours).
- To refer fewer than 6% of infants for follow-up outpatient screening.
- To achieve successful connection on 70% referred for additional evaluation and to document efforts to connect 100% of infants in need of care.
- To refer fewer than 3% of infants for audiologic and medical evaluation.

Figures 6–6A and 6–6B represent the quarterly statistics for the two model UNHS programs. Both programs were able to screen 95% or more of their infants prior to discharge. Both UNHS programs referral rates varied because of addition of screening staff, turnover, and need for instruction of new personnel. Screening equipment, in particular, has a learning curve. It takes time for the screener to acquire expertise at placing the probe into the infant's ear. As the screener becomes more adept at this task, the referral rate decreases. Both UNHS programs more than exceeded the benchmark of the 70% return for follow-up rate.

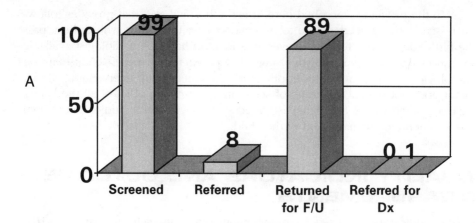

☐ Percentages of Program Quality Indicators

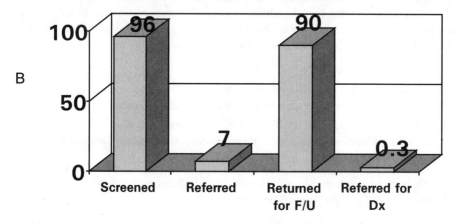

☐ Percentages of Program Quality Indicators

Figure 6-6 Quarterly statistics from DPOAE (A) and TEOAE (B) universal newborn infant hearing screening programs.

SUMMARY

On a monthly basis, the audiologist tracks data and information on all newborns screened to assure that each infant receives the care needed. In addition, program statistics are monitored to assure that the screening program is stable and "in control," to use the language of statistical process control. We learned that yearly and quarterly reviews were ineffective. Too much time elapsed before a problem could be recognized and remedied. UNHS is a new program in our model hospitals. The statistics reflect this but also show continuous improvement over the initial year. Whatever technology, whatever information system, whatever follow-up protocols are in place, continuous improvement is the goal so that each baby detected with hearing loss in our hospitals can obtain the services needed for optimal health and development.

Rose F. Kennedy Center, Albert Einstein College of Medicine: Hearing and Middle Ear Screening for Older Infants and Toddlers

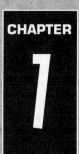

CHAPTER

1

Judith S. Gravel, Ph.D., Janie Chobot, M.S., and Christine Liskow, M.S.

INTRODUCTION

This chapter describes hearing screening procedures used in a pediatric evaluation and rehabilitation program within a large urban medical center. The population described, infants and toddlers from approximately 6 months to 3 years of age, are usually not targeted for large-scale institutional hearing screening because of the need for specialized personnel and instrumentation. Children in this age group are usually seen by an audiologist when parents or caretakers suspect a hearing loss, or when the child is being evaluated for speech, language, or other developmental delays. The assessment described here consists of physiologic and behavioral assessment procedures including visual reinforcement audiometry.

GOALS OF THE SCREENING PROGRAM

The overall mission of the Children's Hearing Program (CHP) of the Children's Evaluation and Rehabilitation Center (CERC) at the Rose F. Kennedy Center is the early detection and management of infants and children with hearing loss and other auditory disorders.

The goal of CHP's screening component is to detect debilitating childhood hearing loss including hearing loss associated with recurrent otitis media with effusion (OME). Because of birth risk, economic, environmental and social stresses, many children are at increased risk not only for peripheral hearing loss, but also for higher-order auditory processing dysfunction. Identification of children with this latter auditory disorder is also a program goal.

SETTING

The CERC was established in 1957, and moved to its present site at the Rose F. Kennedy Center in early 1970. The Kennedy Center is located on the campus of the Jacobi Medical Center (JMC, formerly the Bronx Municipal Hospital Center). The Kennedy Center/JMC complex is adjacent to the campus of the Albert Einstein College of Medicine, Bronx, New York.

CERC is part of a national network of federally funded University Affiliated Programs (UAP) that serve as major training centers for medical and allied health care professions. CERC is one of the largest and most comprehensive facilities of its kind, staffed by over 200 professional and non-professional employees.

The majority of children served by CERC live in the Bronx, a large urban multicultural, ethnically diverse Borough of the City of New York. The population served by CERC is made up primarily (80%) of minority groups who live in poverty or are families of low income. The prevalence of developmental disabilities in the pediatric population served by CERC is higher than average. This is related to the prevalence of factors such as low birth weight, prematurity, maternal drug and alcohol use, HIV infection, reduced access to medical care, adolescent pregnancy, and environmental issues.

Local hospitals, clinics, primary care providers, physicians, schools, day care centers, community agencies, and parents/caregivers refer children to CERC when a developmental disability is suspected. Children are screened at intake and assigned (depending on their suspected disability and age) to one of six multidisciplinary teams. Each CERC team minimally includes a developmental pediatrician, psychologist, and social worker and may also include a speech-language pathologist, psychiatrist, nurse, dentist, physiatrist, physical and occupational therapist, special educator, and learning disability specialist. Audiology services are provided to all teams by CHP. Audiologists attend the various team meetings as necessary. Children referred to CERC receive comprehensive medical and developmental assessment, and, when appropriate, therapeutic intervention and follow-up services. In fiscal year 1997–1998, CERC maintained an active caseload of 7,000 clients who generated more than 50,000 visits during the period. CERC received 2,769 new referrals during 1997–1998, accepted 1,935, and actively followed 10,332 children during the year.

The one audiologic test suite of the Children's Hearing Program used for hearing screening and audiologic assessments is located on the first floor of the Kennedy Center. Following identification and confirmation of an auditory disorder, the management component (the Children's Hearing Intervention Program: CHIP) of CHP provides selection, evaluation, verification and monitoring of amplification devices, direct auditory therapies (aural rehabilitation), parent-child support, liaisons with children's schools, and advocacy services. CHIP services are provided on the fourth floor of the Rousso Annex, which is within a quarter of a mile from the Kennedy Center. In 1998, visits to CHIP totaled 2,856; 1,925 (67%) were for audiologic assessment, and 931 (33%) were for CHIP (hearing aid/aural habilitation) services.

TARGET POPULATION

For the purpose of this report, the target population is young children with various forms of auditory dysfunction who are between 6 and 36 months of age. This target group includes young children with all forms of peripheral hearing loss (cochlear, conductive and mixed), as well as those with neural disorders (auditory neuropathy). Several Kennedy Center, New York City, and New York State programs have affected the composition of this target group, as well as our ability to service these children.

Between 1995 and 1998, the *New York State Department of Health Demonstration Neonatal Hearing Screening Project* funded the development of three universal newborn hearing screening programs at hospitals within our immediate geographical area. These medical facilities (two municipal hospitals and one private) screen the hearing of approximately 10,000 newborns annually. Coverage of the inpatient population at these hospitals has been excellent with approximately 97% of births screened before discharge. Despite our best efforts, as well as the attainment of a low in-hospital refer rate (≤3%), our ability to follow-up the in-hospital "missed" and "referred" infants as out-patients has been low (50% or less in two of the three facilities).

In addition, slightly less than one-half (approximately 9,000) of infants born annually in the Bronx (about 19,000) are born in the remaining four hospitals that currently do not have a universal newborn hearing screening program. For both groups (infants lost to follow-up and unscreened newborns), early identification of hearing loss is delayed until parent or primary care provider concern is raised over hearing ability or communication development.

Infants and young children with OME are a targeted group for early detection of hearing loss. This is because of our long-term experience with the CERC population, as well as ongoing investigations at the Kennedy Center (Clinical Research Center for Communicative Disorders) on the communication and academic sequelae of recurrent OME and hearing loss. A close working relationship with ear, nose, and throat (ENT) physicians in the Department of Otolaryngology has allowed interfacing medical, surgical and audiologic services for infants and toddlers who experience persistent middle ear disorders.

The infants and toddlers with developmental disabilities who are receiving evaluation and intervention through the various CERC multidisciplinary teams are also a CHP target group. These include young children (6–36 months) who have physical disabilities, cognitive disabilities, behavioral problems, HIV infection, learning problems, hearing loss, and speech and language delays.

A recently developed CERC program provides developmental surveillance of graduates of the neonatal intensive care unit (NICU). The goal of the program is the early detection of developmental disabilities in these high-risk infants. Hearing screening is provided by CHP between 6–12 months of age, regardless of the outcome of the newborn hearing screening. NICU graduates at risk for progressive hearing loss or late-onset hearing loss who pass the early hearing test in the first year continue to receive long-term monitoring of their hearing.

New York City's Early Intervention (EI) program has resulted in an increase in referrals to CERC. In 1998, 24% (460) of the new referrals (1,935) to CERC were of children under the age of three years. For infants and toddlers under the age of 18 months, the primary reasons for referrals were 1) global developmental delay and 2) birth-risk factors. Young children over 18 months of age were most often referred to CERC because of speech/language delay. Recently (Spring 1999) a *Clinical Practice Guideline on Assessment and Intervention for Communication Disorders in Young Children* (ages 0–3 years) has been developed and published by the New York State Department of Health. The *Guideline* recommends hearing testing by an audiologist experienced in pediatric assessment be completed as part of the identification and evaluation of young children with suspected or confirmed communication disorders. In addition, the

Guideline recommends ongoing surveillance for progressive and late-onset cochlear hearing loss and conductive hearing loss (secondary to OME). When diagnosed, children with hearing loss are eligible for services through New York City's EI program. We anticipate that the new *Communication Disorders Guideline* will further increase referrals to CERC/CHP for hearing testing in infants and toddlers because of our expertise in pediatric audiologic testing.

SCREENING PERSONNEL

The CHP team is composed of one research audiologist, three clinical audiologists, one pediatric otolaryngologist, a rotating ENT resident, a developmental pediatrician, a child psychologist, and two secretaries. CHP evaluation offers a medical component as well as a planning component in the assessment, education, and habilitation/rehabilitation process of children with confirmed hearing loss/auditory disorders. Only certified and licensed pediatric audiologists conduct hearing screening and audiologic assessments of infants and young children in the targeted population.

INSTRUMENTATION AND TEST PROTOCOL

CERC audiology has one double-wall IAC test booth (control and exam room) that is used for hearing screening and comprehensive audiologic evaluations. Visual reinforcers for both manual and computer-assisted test procedures (see descriptions below) are located in the examination room. The computer controlling IVRA (Intelligent Hearing Systems, Miami, FL), otoacoustic emissions (ILO-88), and middle ear analyzer (Grason-Stadler GSI-33) are located in the control room. In addition, a two-channel clinical audiometer (Grason-Stadler GSI-16) is housed in the control room and located in front of a window between the control and examination rooms. A portable audiometer and speaker/amplifier are located on a small table within the examination room. This is used for manual VRA (one tester). A foot switch located under the audiometer/table controls visual reinforcers associated with the manual VRA method (see below).

TEST METHODS

Screen of Hearing History

At the beginning of an initial assessment, a parent/caretaker is asked four questions: 1) Are there any concerns about speech and language development; 2) Is there a history of otitis media; 3) Are there concerns about responses or inconsistent responses to sound; and, 4) Is there a history of hearing loss in the family? A positive response (yes) to any of the questions raises the index of suspicion regarding the possible presence of hearing loss.

IVRA (Intelligent VRA)—Computer-Assisted Test Procedures

On some occasions the CAST (Classification of Audiograms by Sequential Testing) automated screening algorithm of the three IVRA (Intelligent Visual Reinforcement Audiometry, Intelligent Hearing Systems, Miami, FL) procedures is used to screen infants and young children. CAST is used to provide an overall view of the child's hearing status. CAST screening is completed using sound-field presentation of the test stimuli. CAST patterns 1 and 2 (audiogram with predicted thresholds of 20 dB or better) are used as indicators of a screening "pass." Any other pattern (3–9) results in a manual VRA test session to determine thresholds in sound field at four test frequencies (0.5k, 1k, 2k, and 4k Hz: see below). In addition to CAST screening, tympanometry, middle ear muscle reflex thresholds, and TEOAEs are also obtained. There must be agreement among the tests for the child to be considered a screening "pass." Any discord among measures, indication of unilateral hearing loss of any type, middle ear disorder, or concern expressed by the parent results in threshold measures. Reinforcers are used whether the response is a head turn or play task. The use of CAST in hearing screening of young children is described more thoroughly in Merer and Gravel (1997).

VRA

Our focus at the initial audiologic test is to determine if there is any evidence of a hearing disorder. The IVRA procedure has two algorithms that are suitable for this stage; Optimized Hearing Test Algorithm (OHTA), and the standard 5-up, 5-down threshold search procedure. OHTA is the most commonly used of the IVRA procedures for initial audiologic testing as it provides thresholds at four test frequencies (0.5k, 1k, 2k, and 4k Hz) obtained using an interleaving staircase procedure. OHTA also provides a quantified indicator of test validity (percent response to control trial intervals), as well as a measure of the child's motivation throughout the test session (percent response to probe trials). We also use a manual VRA procedure for audiologic testing.

Regardless of whether an automated or manual VRA test procedure is used, protocols are similar. Multiple visual reinforcers (3 or 4 toy cabinets) are used to reinforce the correct response behavior (head turn/play response during a signal trial).

Initially for infants and toddlers (<24 months) the head-turn response is taught, capitalizing on the child's natural propensity to turn toward (orient to) a novel or interesting sound. At our facility, sound-field presentations of the test stimuli are used. Unless there is information to the contrary, the start level is 30 dBHL at 500 Hz (narrow band of noise or FM tone). If a head turn toward the loudspeaker occurs, the response is reinforced. The signal is presented at the same level a second time regardless of whether or not there was a response to the first. After two presentations, an adaptive procedure is intiated using a 20 dB down, 10 dB up procedure. If there is no response to the 30 dBHL test signal, the presentation level is raised to 50 dBHL and a similar test sequence is initiated. If no response to 70 or 90 dB is observed, sound-field testing is discontinued and the infant or child is taught the response using a bone conducted test signal (250 or 500 Hz at 45 or 55 dBHL, respectively). This provides a salient vibrotactile signal allowing the child to learn the response procedure. Often a 5 dB step size can be used for threshold assessment in this age range. If the infant or child remains motivated after the sound-field thresholds have been obtained, bone conduction testing, followed by individual ear testing is completed.

Reinforcement is provided only after a correct response (head turn when test stimulus is presented). Control trials (silent test intervals) are interspersed (even in the manual procedure) to monitor false positive response behaviors. False positive responding is the greatest danger in VRA assessment. The computer-assisted procedure provides a way of systematically monitoring the false positive rate over the test session, thereby allowing the audiologist to determine the validity of the test results. In manual VRA methods, it is imperative that close attention be paid to the high likelihood that false positive responding by an infant anxious to see the toy reinforcers is providing an inaccurate estimate of hearing thresholds.

A portable audiometer located in the test suite is often used to shape the head turn so that a single audiologist seated in the same room as the child and parent can complete the test. For the IVRA procedure, this is the test arrangement of choice; the audiologist interfaces with the computer via a hand-held response box. For VRA testing, we find the single examiner test method to be highly desirable. The audiologist maintains the child in the midline position (through manipulation of a mildly distracting toy), affects the child's motivation, and determines the optimum time for a test trial to be presented. Visual distractions are minimized in the test room and lights are dimmed to maximize interest in the visual reinforcers. When the one examiner manual method is used, the controls of the audiometer and hand movements of the audiologist are concealed from the child.

If a parent reports the child is under treatment for otitis media with effusion, and/or if flat tympanograms are present, bone conducted presentations are sometimes used to condition the response. Often the responses obtained from a young child with a purely conductive hearing loss are more reliable and the response task appears to be learned more rapidly. Initially, the first signal is delivered at 500 Hz at 30 dBHL; if there is a response to two presentations, the intensity level is lowered to 10 dBHL for the next trials. Two responses at this level are followed by a change in test frequency to 2000 Hz and the same test sequence is followed. After obtaining bone conducted responses at 500 and 2000 Hz at 10 dB, the stimuli are presented by air conduction (sound field). The protocol described above is then used (beginning at 30 dBHL and lowering or raising the test signal by 20 dB dependent upon the response).

Acoustic Immittance and TEOAE Testing

All children receive acoustic immittance testing to assess middle ear function and ipsilateral and contralateral middle ear muscle reflexes. Children also receive TEOAE as a cross-check of the audiometric results (normal hearing versus hearing loss). The outcome from these measures helps to determine if and when a comprehensive audiologic assessment will take place. The results of the comprehensive assessment determine the need for frequency-specific ABR assessment and ENT/medical evaluation.

COSTS/CHARGES

CERC accepts payment from Medicaid and other health insurance programs. Fee for service is on a sliding scale and families are charged based on their ability to pay. Service related income, insurance, Medicaid, and fee for service comprise 65% of our funding. Other funding is provided by New York City and state grants (20%), federal grants (UAP center grant primarily for training) (10%), endowment, private sources, department contracts, and AECOM (Yeshiva University) support (5%). Of our total active caseload, 73.5% have Medicaid insurance, 12% have commercial insurance, 14.3% are self-pay, and 0.2% are covered by the state-aid (Bureau for Handicapped Children) program. On the average, our center receives $168.00 per child for an audiologic test from Medicaid, $15.10 from self-paying families, and $35.16 from all other commercial insurance companies. As an Early Intervention Provider for both evaluation and therapeutic services, we receive $200 per test and $40 per therapy visit on site ($98, if performed at a preschool site). Families needing assistance in transportation to and from Kennedy Center are often provided with tokens, taxi, or ambulette service, depending on need.

COMMUNICATING WITH FAMILIES

A pediatric audiologist is the only person who conveys the audiologic test results to the family. This is typically done immediately after the test session. If the index of suspicion of sensory hearing loss is high after the initial test, extra time is scheduled after the follow-up comprehensive audiologic assessment for counseling purposes. The audiologist supplies telephone numbers so that parents may contact them during or after this period.

The CHIP program is an excellent setting for communicating results to parents. Shortly after the diagnosis of sensory hearing loss has been made, a CHIP appointment is scheduled that lasts at least one hour. Both parents are encouraged to attend; however, most often only the primary caretaker is present. The results and implications of hearing loss, including the child's functional audiogram, type and degree of hearing loss, psychosocial implications of the loss, and communication and educational options, are explained. Handout materials are provided.

FOLLOW-UP/FOLLOW-THROUGH

Depending on the outcome of the initial audiologic test, the follow-up of children proceeds as follows. If the child exhibits normal hearing and no history of OME, a recommendation for monitoring of speech-language milestones is made. If the child exhibits normal to borderline normal behavioral thresholds and middle ear disorder is suspected based on tympanogram and/or middle ear history, then a follow-up test is generally recommended. Repeated concerns regarding hearing (AC and BC tests usually done at follow-up), atypical tympanograms

(>275 daPa tympanometric width and $Y_{TM} < 0.2$), and/or reduced or absent TEOAEs would result in an ENT referral. Any child with hearing loss, non-compliant (flat) tympanograms, absent middle ear muscle reflexes, and absent TEOAEs is scheduled for repeat testing in one month. The primary care provider (or ENT physician) is notified of the results. If follow-up test results are unchanged, and the child is enrolled in CERC, referral for an ENT examination through the CERC program is made.

Any child with hearing loss in one or both ears, normal tympanograms, elevated or absent middle ear muscle reflexes, and absent TEOAEs in one or both ears is scheduled for comprehensive audiologic assessment within a short time period. If results on the follow-up audiologic assessment are consistent with sensory hearing loss in one or both ears, referral for ENT examination and for frequency-specific ABR are made. Services of the CHIP program are explained to the parent and an appointment for CHIP is made immediately. Middle ear function is monitored periodically in all infants and toddlers throughout their enrollment in CHIP. ENT referrals are made promptly, particularly if the young child is a hearing aid user. Audiologic assessments are completed minimally every 3 months in the year following amplification fitting and then every 6 months for children in this age range.

CASE EXAMPLE 1: TYPICAL "PASS"

Infant age 16 months (corrected age of 12 months) was referred because of a history of NICU stay caused by prematurity (gestational age = 30 weeks; birthweight = 1350 grams). The infant was referred because of concerns regarding motor development (a lag in the development of motor milestones).

Thresholds (10 dB step size) were assessed at 500–4000 Hz using a VRA procedure and the test protocol described above. TEOAEs were present at 6 dB S/N at 2k, 3k, and 4k Hz. Tympanograms were normal and ipsilateral middle ear muscle reflexes were present from 500–4000 Hz at 100 dB HL. Speech awareness thresholds were consistent with the pure tone average. There was no history of OME. Based on the results, the infant was considered to have passed the hearing screening, and follow-up audiologic assessment was recommended if the parent or professionals were concerned about hearing in the future.

CASE EXAMPLE 2: TYPICAL "FAIL/REFER"

A mother suspected hearing loss in one of her twins aged 2.5 years. Differences in responses to environmental sounds, voice, and language delay were noted in the little girl compared to her twin brother. The mother sought private ENT consultation. The ENT physician referred the child to Kennedy Center. The child received audiometric testing consisting of a soundfield behavioral audiogram (manual VRA: protocol specified above), and responses (500–4000 Hz) in the severe to profound hearing loss range were obtained. TEOAEs were absent, tympanograms were normal, and middle ear muscle reflexes (500–4000 Hz) were absent in ipsilateral stimulation at equipment limits, bilaterally. She was immediately referred for ABR and enrolled in CHIP. Later frequency-specific ABR thresholds were consistent with profound hearing loss, bilaterally. The toddler returned to CHP for comprehensive audiologic assessment (a behavioral audiogram consisting of bilateral air and bone conduction thresholds, and repeat of the TEOAE, tympanometry, and middle ear muscle reflex measures). Results were similar to the initial tests and supported the presence of bilateral severe to profound cochlear hearing loss, bilaterally. The toddler was enrolled in CHIP for parent counseling, hearing aid selection, and evaluation and auditory training three times per week. Loaner hearing aids were provided until personal aids were fitted. She was subsequently enrolled in an educational program (oral/aural method) with assistance of a CHIP audiologist in the development of her Individualized Family Service Plan. She is awaiting an FM system through the early intervention system based on CHIP recommendation. Her twin received audiologic assessment during the follow-up and was found to have hearing within normal limits, bilaterally.

SUMMARY

This chapter described hearing screening procedures applicable to infants and toddlers from approximately 6 months to 3 years of age, as used in a pediatric evaluation program affiliated within a large urban medical center. The assessment procedures advocated include a combination of physiologic and behavioral assessment procedures performed by an audiologist. The importance of follow-up and careful communication with families was emphasized.

REFERENCE

Merer, D. M., & Gravel, J. S. (1997). Screening infants and children for hearing loss: An examination of the CAST procedure. *Journal of the American Academy of Audiology, 8*(4), 233–242.

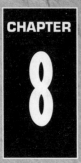

CHAPTER

8

The Chapel Hill-Carrboro (NC) Schools: Hearing and Middle Ear Screening for Preschool and School-Age Children

Martha R. Mundy, Au.D.

INTRODUCTION

Recent decades have seen many changes in the procedures, protocols, and instrumentation used in school-age hearing screening programs. In the mid-1960s, attention was devoted to various methods of group screening in the unfulfilled hope that accurate methods could be developed to allow simultaneous testing of several children by a single examiner. The early 1960s also witnessed the clinical benefits of acoustic impedance measurements, but tympanometry was still not in widespread clinical use a decade later. Today, numerous manufacturers have portable systems, and the addition of acoustic immittance to school hearing screening programs permits identification of otitis media as well as hearing loss.

The school-based hearing screening program described here has been in operation for five years. The program operates under a contractual arrangement between the University of North Carolina and the Chapel Hill–Carrboro City School District, which includes 13 schools and nine Head Start preschool programs. The total enrollment, including preschools, is approximately 9,200. Screening is provided to approximately 2,200 children, mostly at the preschool and elementary levels. Audiologic support services for children with identified hearing loss is provided at all grade levels. The contract for educational audiology services includes school-based and clinic-based services. The bulk of these services are provided during the fall semester.

In school settings, much of the audiology service must occur within the first few months of the school year. Although many schools have speech-language pathologists on-site, educational audiologists, where available, usually cover several schools if not entire districts. A contractual arrangement with a clinical program that employs several audiologists allows flexibility based on the concentrated needs of the fall semester. The student census for the school-age children in our district includes 8 elementary schools, 3 middle schools, and 2 high schools. Three off-site preschool programs and 5 Head Start programs housed within elementary schools are also included. Elementary school screening typically involves 24 on-site days and approximately 2,400 total screenings. Head Start screenings involve eight on-site days.

Our program, like many, is continuously undergoing change. At this time, screening is administered and directly supervised by an audiologist with assistance provided by graduate students in speech-language pathology at elementary schools, and with the assistance of audiology graduate students at Head Start preschools. The model could be replicated with other personnel; however, the direct participation and supervision of an audiologist is essential. The primary goals are identification and referral of hearing loss and otitis media, in a timely and cost-effective manner. Our aim is to have all preschool and elementary school first and second level screenings completed and referrals to parents made by the end of November. This goal has been achieved each year using the procedures described in this chapter.

WHERE TO PERFORM HEARING SCREENING

Among the greatest challenges to the implementation of a hearing screening program for preschool and school-age children is working within the school environment. The first and most obvious obstacle is the inevitable presence of background noise. One might assume that newer buildings would offer a more acceptable hearing screening environment, but newer structures often have centrally located heating and air conditioning systems that cannot be controlled within the space available for screening. When outside temperatures require the operation of these systems, failure rates, especially at lower frequencies, are often higher.

Competing noise is not the only challenge. Space is in tremendous demand for most school environments and not easily relinquished. The program described here requires the presence of the hearing screening team on two school days for the first level screen and one half to one day for the second level rescreen. For the individuals working in a school on a daily basis, the fall is a busy time and the accommodations needed for successful hearing screening compete with other activities. Only after a screening program has been in place for an extended period of time do school staff members understand the necessity of securing a quiet, functional workspace. The location of this space will vary, even within the same school system. Our program has used space in trailers, small conference rooms in the library, and empty classrooms.

It is important to be responsive to the needs of the school and, ultimately, for each school to become responsive to the needs of the screening program. If noise levels in screening areas are excessive, pass/fail criteria must not be altered. We have found it helpful on occasion to provide schools with referral data by grade for children with normal tympanograms. When these numbers are unusually high, it is an objective indicator of the need to provide more favorable conditions. This information, in conjunction with requests for suitable space, helps school administrators understand the importance of the screening environment.

A contact person at each school is necessary to determine the environment available for screening. The room must be large enough to accommodate a group of children and examiners. A small quiet space is more desirable than a large space near high traffic areas. In our program, entire kindergarten, first, and second grade classrooms are brought together to the screening site where four tables (or stations) are set up for testing. We use three separate stations for pure tone audiometry and one for otoscopy and tympanometry. Desks or other furniture are moved from the center of the room and the children sit on the floor while they are given group instruction. If the space available is too small to accommodate an entire class, children are brought in smaller groups while the rest of the class waits nearby, usually in a hallway.

WHEN TO PERFORM HEARING SCREENING

The hearing-screening calendar for the academic year will be determined by examiner availability and school schedules. The first level screening requires two school days for most elementary schools and the second level visit is scheduled 4 to 6 weeks later. School districts have generally established the academic calendar for the following year by late spring. In addition to noting teacher work days and holidays, inquiries need to be made about other activities occurring on scheduled days. These may include but are not limited to schoolwide carnivals, field trips, other screenings (such as dental or vision), and schoolwide academic testing.

Setting the schedule for the day of the screening also requires the assistance of a school-based contact person to facilitate scheduling of individual classes. A form with 30 minute appointment slots is provided to the contact person for routing to kindergarten, first, and second grade teachers. Any open appointment slots are used for scheduling third, fourth, and fifth graders who are due for re-evaluation, are being referred for educational testing, or for whom parents or teachers have expressed concerns. Recently, this has been accomplished with support from school principals at early staff meetings. Asking teachers to select a 30 minute time block during faculty meetings is ideal because their class day is not interrupted and they can choose times that do not conflict with lunch or special activities. Because the initial screening generally occurs on two separate days, field trips and other planned absences can be avoided. Kindergarten classes are screened early in the day to avoid conflicts with lunch schedules and the subsequent 'quiet' or nap times that often occur after lunch in preschools and lower grade levels. A 30 minute block of time is sufficient for most classes of 25 students, using three testing stations, with time remaining for many first and second grade classes.

Scheduling second level retests for children who do not pass the initial screening is more complicated. Usually only two or three children will be identified from each class, so children from several classes share a time slot. Since all of these children are being rescreened, additional time must be allowed for otoscopy and tympanometry. Additional time is also necessary to allow for pure tone screening. Sweep frequency screening usually takes longer because of a higher proportion of children who will not pass and because of the additional noise generated by groups of children from different classes arriving at varying times. The schedule is arranged so that 10 to 15 children arrive in a 30 minute time slot, depending on grade level. Because the second screening involves only a few children from each class, times are assigned and teachers are notified with the understanding that they may request rescheduling.

Screening needs that arise after the scheduled visits in the fall are handled by school-based speech-language pathologists or school nurses. This becomes necessary in the case of children who are absent or enrolled after screening is completed. Thus, in-service training of school personnel by the consulting audiologist is an important part of the contractual arrangement.

TARGET POPULATIONS

Children are targeted for screening based on the goals of the screening program; requirements the school must follow in re-evaluating certain children; resources of the school to support a screening program; and other community programs that may offer hearing screening. Our target populations include:

- Mass screening of Head Start and school-based pre-kindergarten classes, kindergarten, first and second grade;
- Individual screening of children (third through twelfth grade) whose names are on a "watch" list as a result of referrals from previous screenings;
- Individual children (third through twelfth grade) who are being evaluated for special services eligibility;
- Individual children (third through twelfth grade) for whom teachers or parents have expressed concern.

Obtaining student names via class lists prior to the scheduled screening day is essential. We have found it time-consuming and disruptive to complete forms while children are waiting. A little experience with shy kindergartners quickly confirms the benefit of having a closed set of names provided in advance. Teacher provided nametags for younger students are especially helpful. Class lists can be obtained from attendance rosters at each elementary school and transferred onto screening forms. A more expeditious way of transferring names onto screening forms is to request a systemwide listing from the general administration's school registrar. These are loaded into a database, which can sort data and generate reports by school, classroom teacher, and grade (Figure 8–1). Because the first month of school is a busy time for school personnel, it is imperative that these arrangements be discussed and agreed upon well in advance.

SCREENING PERSONNEL

The validity of the program rests solidly upon the individuals who conduct the screening. These individuals are often parent volunteers, graduate students, or speech-language pathologists; each group has its advantages. Parents bring prior experience with young children, while graduate students often have previous screening experience as well as motivation to fulfill practicum requirements and obtain career competencies. Speech pathologists bring knowledge and experience, but will not have sufficient time available unless this activity is included in their job descriptions. Regardless of who performs the screening, it is essential that the program be conducted under the careful supervision of an audiologist. As noted above, our program uses graduate students in speech-language pathology and audiology who conduct the screening under the direct supervision of an audiologist. An overview of the screening program is provided in early fall

CHCCS Hearing and Middle Ear Screening Program

School: Lincoln   Grade: K   Home Room: Hubbard

	Pure Tone Results						Tympanometry				Otoscopy	
	Right			Left			Right		Left		Right	Left
	1000	2000	4000	1000	2000	4000	Ytm	MEP	Ytm	MEP		

Andrews, Donald
08/30/2000 — Right: + + + Left: + + + | Tympanometry R: -200 L: Ad | Otoscopy R: L:

Bailey, Philip
08/30/2000 — Right: + + + Left: + + . + | Tympanometry R: Pass Pass L: Pass Pass | Otoscopy R: L:

Chu, Jill
08/30/2000 — Right: + + + Left: + + + | Tympanometry R: Pass Pass L: Pass Pass | Otoscopy R: L:

Cook, Mary
08/30/2000 — Right: + + + Left: + + + | Tympanometry R: -175 L: -200 | Otoscopy R: ok L: ok

Daly, John
08/30/2000 — Right: + + + Left: + + + | Tympanometry R: Pass Pass L: Pass Pass | Otoscopy R: L:

Irving, Carol
08/30/2000 — Right: + + + Left: + + + | Tympanometry R: Pass Pass L: Pass Pass | Otoscopy R: L:

Jones, Elizabeth
08/30/2000 — Right: + + + Left: + + + | Tympanometry R: L: | Otoscopy R: L:

Kilpatrick, Ann
08/30/2000 — Right: + + + Left: + + + | Tympanometry R: -175 L: -200 | Otoscopy R: L:

Larson, Kim
08/30/2000 — Right: + + + Left: 25 + + | Tympanometry R: Flat L: Pass Pass | Otoscopy R: OK L: OK

Lee, Carson
08/30/2000 — Right: + + + Left: + + 25 | Tympanometry R: Pass Pass L: .2 | Otoscopy R: OK L: CNS-debris

Figure 8-1 Display of database for CHCCS hearing and middle ear screening program (names shown are fictitious).

and a notebook with relevant information (protocols, schedules, directions to schools) is available for reference. In addition, essential elements are reviewed on the day of screening before the first class arrives: equipment operation, earphone placement, listening checks, and recording of test data.

INSTRUMENTATION FOR HEARING SCREENING

Portable pure tone air conduction audiometers are essential in any screening program. In our district, all schools have a single channel portable audiometer on site for occasional hearing screening by the speech-language pathologist or the school nurse. Audiometers are calibrated annually during the summer and listening checks are conducted prior to each use. On the day of the screening, the team brings two additional portable audiometers in order to provide three screening stations. In general, supra-aural earphones are used rather than insert earphones to improve efficiency and reduce cost. Our experience has been that most preschool and kindergarten children readily accept earphones, although play procedures are often needed at pre-kindergarten levels. Table 8–1 provides a list of equipment and supplies required for each site.

TEST PROTOCOL

Hearing is screened at 20 dBHL at 1000, 2000, and 4000 Hz. A positive response to at least two presentations for each ear at each frequency is required for a child to pass. A supervising audiologist is on site and present during all testing. When a student does not respond at 20 dBHL, the examiner increases the intensity in 10 dB steps until a response is observed. If a response is observed at 30 dBHL, they return to the screening level and provide another opportunity at 20 dBHL. This information is used to determine which children are to be

---

TABLE 8-1 Equipment and supplies needed for hearing and middle ear screening in a school or preschool setting.

Portable audiometers

Toys for play audiometry

Extension cords and power strips

Tympanometers

Eartips for tympanometry probe

Otoscopes and specula

Disinfectant for specula and eartips

Surgical gloves and alcohol wipes

Portable filebox containing:

    Class lists and screening forms, presorted for each day

    Referral forms

    Handouts for parents and teachers

Loose-leaf notebook containing:

    Referral log for each school

    Complete screening schedule

    List of students on watch list or identified by school personnel

    Original of each form

rescreened in 4–6 weeks and which should be referred immediately. The screening form is used to record each response. If the student does not respond, the lowest response level is recorded. Examiners do not conduct formal threshold determination procedures, but are instructed to find a minimal response level when the child does not detect the 20 dBHL screening stimulus (see Figure 8–1). Any child who does not pass the pure tone screen is seen during the same session for otoscopy and tympanometry. Children who have normal tympanograms but do not pass the initial hearing screening are tested again at another station. We have found that this immediate second test at the first level screening eliminates many unnecessary referrals and rechecks at the second screening.

Tympanometry is performed on all children only for preschool and kindergarten classes, where children are screened with both pure tones and tympanometry. Children with abnormally low static admittance (≤ 0.1 mmho) suggestive of otitis media with effusion (OME) are usually seen again at the second level rescreen (in 4–6 weeks). When there is evidence of acute OME from otoscopy or behavioral indicators, an immediate medical referral is made. Immediate referral is also made in cases of abnormally large equivalent volume estimates accompanied by flat tympanograms (in the absence of tympanostomy tubes), indicating possible tympanic membrane perforation. These children are also seen again at the second screening visit. Abnormal tympanograms are always repeated. We have noted that occasionally while using handheld instruments, tympanograms may initially be flat with normal equivalent volume, but normal when repeated. We have also noted that some children have tympanometric patterns that do not warrant medical referral (e.g., negative tympanometric peak pressure) but do not pass the hearing screening. These children are seen again at the second level rescreening visit. It should be noted that our referral criteria differ somewhat from those recommended by ASHA (1997). Abnormal tympanometric width, in our experience, occurs infrequently. The most common abnormalities are reduced static admittance (flat tympanograms of .0 or .1 mmho) and negative pressure.

FORMS AND PAPERWORK

After testing is complete for a given class, screening data are reviewed and results transferred to a master form for each class (Figure 8–2). The raw data obtained on the original screening forms signed by each examiner are retained but not distributed to the school, since each form has only partial data. Three copies of the master forms are made at the end of the screening day. The audiologist keeps the originals and the copies are left with the school liaison, who distributes copies to other school personnel involved in the screening program. Those individuals vary among schools but may include the speech-language pathologist, school nurses, or special education personnel. In addition, screening results are transferred to the students' "health cards." In our district, health cards are pulled from each student's cumulative record at the beginning of the year and filed by class for easier access during screening and other health related school activities. Results of pure tone audiometry and tympanometry are recorded

CHCCS Hearing Screening Summary

School Franklin   **Grade** K   **Home Room** Sheffler

Name	Test Date	HealthCard	Disposition
Andrews, David	09/01/2000	☑	Pass
Bartlett, John	09/01/2000	☑	Pass
Catlett, Elizabeth	09/01/2000	☑	Pass
Davis, Kiesha	09/01/2000	☑	Pass
Gatewood, Dennis	09/01/2000	☐	Absent
Grant, Amy	09/01/2000	☑	Pass
Jin, Lu	09/01/2000	☑	Pass
Padrovia, Andrei	09/01/2000	☑	Pass
Rogers, Tyrone	09/01/2000	☐	Pass
Stevens, Kelly	09/01/2000	☑	Pass
Thomas, Arthur	09/01/2000	☑	Pass
Villanova, Andre	09/01/2000	☑	Pass
Weston, Thomas	09/01/2000	☐	Pass
Youngblood, Sarah	09/01/2000	☐	Pass
Zanzot, David	09/01/2000	☑	Pass

Tuesday, September 05, 2000   Page 1 of 2

Figure 8-2 CHCCS Hearing Screening Summary for a portion of one class (names shown are fictitious).

along with the date and the audiologist's initials. Occasionally, referral decisions are altered when recording individual data onto health cards. For example, a student who did not pass the hearing screening, with borderline results for both ears and borderline tympanograms (e.g., 0.2 mmho static admittance), may have been put on a recheck list for the second level follow-up screen. In the process of recording information onto the health card, however, it may be clear that this student has a history of failed screenings with borderline results. In that case, a referral would be made after the first level screen for a complete audiologic evaluation. In such cases, teacher input regarding academic performance is sometimes requested using the SIFTER (Screening Instrument for Targeting Educational Risk; Anderson, 1989).

REFERRALS AND COMMUNICATION WITH PARENTS

Screening programs will fall short of their intended goals if mechanisms are not in place to ensure that parents understand the screening results and recommendations. Unfortunately, the goal of keeping parents informed is often in conflict with the goal of maintaining efficiency and cost effectiveness. Multipurpose forms can aid in reducing some of the attendant chaos of paperwork often found at the end of a screening day. Because many families wanted additional information at the time of referral, parent notification has evolved from simple form letters to more detailed all-purpose forms with checklists (see Appendix 8–A through 8–D). These forms can be easily supplemented with "Parent Notes" providing additional information not conveyed in the standard notification forms. Or they can be sent in lieu of medical or audiologic referral when a student passes pure tone screening but has abnormal tympanograms, or when substantial (but non-occluding) cerumen remains. In these notes, parents are encouraged to contact their primary care providers to determine if medical management is recommended. A telephone number where parents can contact the school audiologist is noted on all forms.

For many families, information regarding hearing loss or a middle ear disorder comes as no surprise. Often these children have a longstanding history of otitis media, and in such cases a relationship already exists with the child's medical provider. For other families, however, obtaining medical examination and treatment is an enormous challenge. School personnel are needed to facilitate follow-up evaluations with families who have transportation problems, lack information regarding medical resources, or have limited fluency in English. Consequently, all forms describing screening outcomes are given to the school liaison who distributes them to the student's family. The school liaison then informs families of available community resources for obtaining medical evaluations and, as needed, assists them with transportation to medical or audiologic evaluations.

MEDICAL REFERRAL

Referrals for medical treatment are made when tympanograms are abnormal on rescreening, when hearing loss persists, or when otoscopic inspection suggests excessive cerumen, the presence of a foreign body, or evidence of ear disease. Medical intervention generally occurs promptly when hearing loss is clearly demonstrated or when tympanograms are consistent with OME. For example, during the past screening year, four children with 35–45 dB conductive hearing losses were seen within one month of the screening referral by ENT physicians who subsequently scheduled the children for placement of tympanostomy tubes. In other cases, however, the medical follow-up examination may conflict with the results provided by the school screening. This is unavoidable when hearing loss or middle ear dysfunction has resolved in the interval from referral to examination. More frequently, however, parents receive conflicting information because of different perspectives on what is normal and what constitutes a hearing loss. The audiometric criterion of 0–25 dBHL has a long history of use in defining normal hearing. More recently, 0–15 dBHL has been advocated by audiologists as a more appropriate range of normal hearing for children, based on studies that have indicated delays in speech, language, or educational achievement, even for mild degrees of hearing loss.

The medical perspective on the child with OME generally includes consideration of educational impact, but is fundamentally concerned with physical health. If the child without a history of frequent acute episodes of OME has hearing levels of 30 dBHL or better, the physician may well adopt a plan of watchfulness rather than recommending pharmacological or surgical intervention. In such cases, accommodations for children with "minimal hearing loss" may need to occur in the school arena, with non-medical interventions such as sound-field FM, which we have found to be an especially viable option for children at lower elementary levels. Medical management can involve a lengthy observation period to allow a non-acute condition to resolve and observation may encompass a significant part of the academic year. When children have documented histories of hearing loss and are eligible for special education services, appropriate amplification systems can often be provided by the school district.

When hearing is within normal range but tympanograms continue to be abnormal, a note describing tympanometry is sent home and parents are encouraged to contact their primary care providers for guidance about follow-up. It is our practice to provide parents with information about middle ear status and to place those children on a watch list for rescreens and evidence of educational risk (using the SIFTER).

AUDIOLOGIC REFERRAL

As previously noted, hearing is considered a pass on pure tones if a response is obtained at 1000, 2000, and 4000 Hz for each ear at 20 dBHL. Nine children with unilateral sensorineural loss have been identified during the past four academic years, based on screening failure at only one frequency in one ear. Bilateral hearing loss requiring amplification will usually have been identified prior to school age, but not always. Five children with bilateral loss have been identified by the screening program over the past four years. The children with bilateral hearing loss are now fitted with acoustic amplification and FM systems. The children with unilateral hearing loss are being closely followed; some use assistive listening devices on a selective basis.

COSTS/CHARGES

Financing of this program is accomplished through a contractual arrangement between the school district and the University. The contract has three components: 1) hearing/middle ear screening, which accounts for about 50% of the time/resources committed to the educational audiology contract, 2) diagnostic testing/follow-up for children referred from the screening program, which accounts for about 25% of resource allocation, and 3) general audiology services to children identified as deaf or hard-of-hearing, which accounts for the remaining 25% of resource allocation. A group rate is negotiated for the screening component; the other two components are billed on an hourly basis.

In our program, mass screening occurs only in the elementary schools and Head Start preschools. An additional seven on-site days involve screening middle and high school children who are being re-evaluated for special services eligibility. Unless additional financial resources are added as the district expands, additional screening sites cannot be added without sacrificing services to deaf and hard-of-hearing students already identified. Whether the audiology services are delivered via contract or by an individual employed by the school district, the hours available for screening are limited. Time must be available to provide follow-up for children already identified.

Several changes to this program have been made in recent years to improve efficiency without compromising our fundamental goals. First, we have reduced the size of the population targeted for mass screening. As shown in Table 8–2, the number of children who pass the initial hearing screen increases with age. Since our goals include the identification of children with chronic or recurrent OME, eliminating younger age groups where OME is more prevalent would be counterproductive. However, examination of third grade class lists and outcomes revealed that the prevalence of OME was too low to provide a sufficient number of referrals to justify the time and expense incurred. Furthermore, we discovered that most of the third graders who did not pass would have been identified by a "watch list" from the second grade roster. In other words, all third graders who persisted with OME continued to be affected when they were in second grade, and thus could be identified for further screening on that basis. Consequently, mass screening of third grade classrooms has been eliminated.

Other changes have involved eliminating routine hearing screening for middle and high school students new to the district, although entering students

TABLE 8-2 Screening outcomes on first screen, in a typical school year, using a combination of pure tone screening and acoustic immittance (static admittance and equivalent volume).

GRADE	N	Pass on First Screen (%)
Head Start and Preschool	128	81
Kindergarten	644	93
First grade	553	96
Second grade	627	98
Overall	1,952	95

with active Individualized Education Plans (IEPs) have hearing screening conducted by their speech-language pathologist. Despite concerns about the increasing prevalence of noise-induced hearing loss in teenagers, our observations have not confirmed this. In fact, pass rates have consistently been at or near 100% at the middle and high school for students not receiving special services. This finding could be due to the fact that relatively few students in this age range are tested. Instead of mass hearing screening, an informational program to promote hearing conservation among these students would be a more appropriate first step. Screening in conjunction with such an informational program would combine the best of prevention and identification. Attempts are underway to implement such a program in the less hectic spring semester.

UNRESOLVED ISSUES AND FUTURE DIRECTIONS

Computerized Tracking

Pilot testing is now underway with a system we created in Microsoft Access to generate summary reports and facilitate tracking of referral outcomes. In addition to improving communication among the audiologist, school nurses, and parents, computerization of the screening program is making it easier to generate the data we need to evaluate the performance of our screening protocols.

Instrumentation and Methodology

Although not previously implemented in this program, a future modification under consideration is the utilization of insert earphones for second level screenings. This would allow for greater attenuation of room noise and would avoid over-referrals caused by poor headphone placement. The cost for disposable eartips would be considerably less for the number of children seen for rescreens and thus more easily justifiable.

We are also considering implementation of otoacoustic emissions. The advent of portable, battery-operated, and relatively inexpensive otoacoustic emissions screeners have facilitated their use in school screening programs. The benefits are obvious for those children who are difficult to test because of developmental delays or lack of cooperation. The widespread use of OAEs as the first level screen to identify hearing loss and middle ear disease has promise, but requires further study. We recently participated in a multi-site investigation exploring the efficacy of OAEs for school-based hearing and middle ear screening. Findings for our cohort suggested good agreement between emission screening and pure tone/tympanometric screening (Christensen, 2000).

Intervention

Medical intervention is not necessarily the only option for children with mild or fluctuating hearing loss secondary to OME. Even when medical intervention is obtained and hearing levels return to normal, the child's past history of poor hearing may remain a factor. There is some evidence that children with histories of chronic or recurrent hearing loss secondary to otitis media continue to experience difficulty with auditory processing, even when hearing sensitivity returns to normal. Non-medical interventions such as sound-field FM, although usually obtained for a specific student, are beneficial to other students in the classroom as well. Although the benefit of such technology has been demonstrated anecdotally, school systems often resist purchase of these systems on a districtwide basis. This is caused, in part, by the budgetary divide between monies available for improving school facilities and those allocated for student services where the purchase of such equipment has traditionally originated. Recent recommendations for the development of standards for classroom acoustics may change this. The Access Board, the agency that assures compliance with the Americans with Disabilities Act, was recently petitioned by the parent of a child with sensorineural hearing loss to develop minimum standards for classroom acoustics. Standards are currently being drafted.

SUMMARY

There are many components to a successful school-based screening program. Equipment must be properly selected and maintained, personnel must be well qualified, procedures and protocols must be established, and record keeping must be carefully maintained. In addition, screening and referral outcomes must be closely monitored and used for continuous improvement. This activity is time intensive and demanding, but the rewards are many. Timely identification and management of hearing loss and middle ear disease assures each child the opportunity to maximize his or her educational and social opportunities during the critical preschool and school-age years.

References

American Speech-Language Hearing Association. (1997). Guidelines for audiologic screening. Rockville, MD: ASHA. ISBN: 0-910329-96-6.

Anderson, K. (1989). *Screening Instrument for Targeting Educational Risk*. Little Rock, AR: The Educational Audiology Association.

Christensen, L. (2000). The use of otoacoustic emissions for school-age and adult populations. Presented at the annual convention of the American Academy of Audiology, Chicago, IL, March 2000.

APPENDIX 8-A

REPORT TO PARENTS ABOUT HEARING SCREENING
HEARING EVALUATION RECOMMENDED

STUDENT: SCHOOL/TEACHER: DATE:

Your child's hearing was screened today at school.

PURE-TONE TESTING suggests a hearing decrease in the RIGHT/LEFT/BOTH ears. Results are recorded below:

	1000 Hz	2000 Hz	4000 Hz
RIGHT			
LEFT			

This is consistent with: _____ hearing decrease for the RIGHT ear, and _____ hearing decrease for the LEFT ear.

TYMPANOMETRY is a test that provides information about how well the eardrum accepts sound. When tympanograms are "flat" there is often fluid behind the eardrum. Your child's tympanograms were normal for the RIGHT/LEFT/BOTH ears.

	Type	Equivalent Volume	Other Comments
RIGHT			
LEFT			

OTOACOUSTIC EMISSIONS are done when students do not pass the pure tone screening and have normal tympanograms. This test measures a faint echo (emission) created by the inner ear in response to certain sounds. When the emission is present, it confirms normal function within the inner ear (cochlea). When it is absent further evaluation is needed.

	PASS @ 2, 3, 4 kHz	ABSENT @ 2, 3, 4 kHz	Other
RIGHT			
LEFT			

Based on these findings, we recommend that your child be seen for a complete hearing evaluation. Since this recommendation is the result of the school screening program, there is NO CHARGE to families when the evaluation is performed at the Division of Speech and Hearing Sciences Clinic (966-1006) at UNC. If you prefer to have your child evaluated elsewhere, you will be responsible for any charges. If your child is seen at another clinic, please ask the clinician testing your child to complete the back of this form and send the results to the address indicated.

If you think you will have difficulty scheduling or taking your child for evaluation, please contact the school Family Specialist.

Thank you,

Martha R. Mundy, Au.D. (966-1006)
Audiologist

171

APPENDIX 8-B

REPORT TO PARENTS ABOUT HEARING SCREENING
HEARING EVALUATION RECOMMENDED

STUDENT: SCHOOL/TEACHER: DATE:

Your child's hearing was screened today at school. All children in Kindergarten, First, and Second grade have their hearing checked. Some 3RD, 4TH, and 5TH graders are also tested. Students who do not pass the first time and do not appear to have ear disease are retested in four to six weeks to see if their hearing has improved. Today was the SECOND time your child was screened. Results are recorded below:

PURE-TONE TESTING ON _____ suggested a hearing decrease in the RIGHT/LEFT/BOTH ears.

	1000 Hz	2000 Hz	4000 Hz
RIGHT			
LEFT			

PURE-TONE TESTING TODAY suggests a hearing decrease in the RIGHT/LEFT/BOTH ears.

	1000 Hz	2000 Hz	4000 Hz
RIGHT			
LEFT			

Today's results are consistent with: _____ hearing decrease for the RIGHT ear, and _____ hearing decrease for the LEFT ear.

TYMPANOMETRY is a test that provides information about how well the eardrum accepts sound. When tympanograms are "flat," there is often fluid behind the eardrum. This is a common condition during early childhood but not a normal condition for the ears. When fluid is present, infection may be present. Many ears with middle ear fluid, however, are NOT infected. **OTOSCOPY** is the visual inspection of the ear canal and eardrum. Results of tympanometry and otoscopic inspection for your child are:

1ST ( )	Type	Equivalent Volume	Comments	Otoscopy
RIGHT				
LEFT				
TODAY'S				
RIGHT				
LEFT				

Based on these findings, we recommend that your child be seen for a complete hearing evaluation. Since this recommendation is the result of the school-screening program, there is NO CHARGE to families when the evaluation is performed at the Division of Speech and Hearing Sciences Clinic (966-1006) at UNC. If you prefer to have your child evaluated elsewhere, you will be responsible for any charges. If your child is seen at another clinic, please ask the clinician testing your child to complete the back of this form and send the results to the address indicated. If you think you will have difficulty scheduling or taking your child for evaluation, please contact the school Family Specialist.

Martha R. Mundy, Au.D. (966-1006)
Audiologist

APPENDIX 8-C

REPORT TO PARENTS ABOUT HEARING SCREENING
MEDICAL EVALUATION RECOMMENDED

STUDENT: SCHOOL/TEACHER: DATE:

Your child's hearing was screened today at school.

PURE-TONE TESTING suggests a hearing decrease in the RIGHT/LEFT/BOTH ears. Results are recorded below:

	1000 Hz	2000 Hz	4000 Hz
RIGHT			
LEFT			

This is consistent with: _____ hearing decrease for the RIGHT ear, and _____ hearing decrease for the LEFT ear.

TYMPANOMETRY is a test that provides information about how well the eardrum accepts sound. When tympanograms are "flat," there is often fluid behind the eardrum. This is a common condition during childhood but not a normal condition for the ears. When there is fluid behind the eardrum it may or may not be infected. Your child's tympanograms were:

	Type	Equivalent Volume	Comments
RIGHT			
LEFT			

OTOSCOPY is the visual inspection of the ear canal and eardrum. Results of otoscopic inspection for your child are:

	Wax	Appearance	Other
RIGHT			
LEFT			

Based on these findings, we recommend that your child be seen by his/her physician as soon as possible for medical evaluation of the ears. If you will have difficulty scheduling a medical evaluation for your child, please contact the Family Specialist at your child's school. Please ask your physician to complete the reverse of this form and return it to the address indicated.

Thank you,

Martha R. Mundy, Au.D. (966-1006)
Audiologist

APPENDIX 8-D

REPORT TO PARENTS ABOUT HEARING SCREENING
MEDICAL EVALUATION RECOMMENDED

STUDENT: _____

SCHOOL/TEACHER: _____   DATE: _____

Your child's hearing was screened today at school. All children in Kindergarten, First and Second grade have their hearing checked. Some 3rd, 4th, and 5th graders are also tested. Students who do not pass the first time and do not appear to have ear disease are retested in four to six weeks to see if their hearing has improved. Today was the SECOND time your child was screened. Results are recorded below:

PURE-TONE TESTING ON _____ suggested a hearing decrease in the RIGHT/LEFT/BOTH ears.

	1000 Hz	2000 Hz	4000 Hz
RIGHT			
LEFT			

PURE-TONE TESTING TODAY suggests a hearing decrease in the RIGHT/LEFT/BOTH ears.

	1000 Hz	2000 Hz	4000 Hz
RIGHT			
LEFT			

Today's results are consistent with: _____ hearing decrease for the RIGHT ear, and _____ hearing decrease for the LEFT ear.

TYMPANOMETRY is a test that provides information about how well the eardrum accepts sound. When tympanograms are "flat," there is often fluid behind the eardrum. This is a common condition during childhood, but not a normal condition for the ears. When fluid is present, infection may be present. Many ears with middle ear fluid, however, are NOT infected. **OTOSCOPY** is the visual inspection of the ear canal and eardrum. Results of tympanometry and otoscopic inspection for your child are:

1ST ( )	Type	Equivalent Vol.	Comments	Otoscopy
RIGHT				
LEFT				
TODAY'S				
RIGHT				
LEFT				

Based on these findings, we recommend that your child be seen by his/her physician for medical evaluation of the ears. Hearing should be rechecked at the completion of any medical treatment. If you think you will have difficulty scheduling this evaluation for your child, please contact the Family Specialist at your child's school. Please ask your physician to complete the reverse of this form and return it to the address indicated. Follow-up hearing evaluation can be scheduled at NO CHARGE by calling 966-1006.

Thank you,

Martha R. Mundy, Au.D. (966-1006)
Audiologist

Part III: Referral, Follow-Up, and Parent-Professional Communication

INTRODUCTION

Although the identification process has been the primary focus of this text, each author has emphasized the importance of referral and follow-up. In Part III of this text, practitioners from the first state in the United States to engage in universal infant hearing screening, describe the many components of a comprehensive statewide plan. The book concludes with a brief epilogue, giving final emphasis to the importance of skillful and sensitive communication with families.

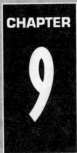

Referral and Follow-Up: The Rhode Island Experience

Ellen Kurtzer-White, M.S.
Mary Jane Johnson, M.Ed.

INTRODUCTION

Rhode Island has the advantage of being somewhat of a microcosm. Traveling from border to border generally requires no more than an hour's drive (with the exception of Block Island, accessible only by boat or air). There is one major metropolitan city, Providence, which is the central location for pediatric medical care and hospitals, state departments of health and education, as well as the state's school for the deaf and hearing center. Women and Infants Hospital, the primary birthing hospital, where the majority of the state's infants are born, is also located in Providence. Given these demographics, Rhode Island was able to successfully pilot a Maternal and Child Health investigation of the feasibility and efficacy of universal neonatal hearing screening. Indeed, the success of the project promulgated legislation in 1993 mandating universal newborn hearing screening, and put Rhode Island at the vanguard of a national trend. Since the law's enactment, 99% of the state's newborns (14,000 annually) have their hearing screened. As of January, 1998, more than 63,000 infants have participated and 2 to 3 per thousand have been identified with varying degrees of permanent hearing loss. In contrast to the 1996 U.S. average age of 30 months, Rhode Island's average age of diagnosis is 3.5 months.

As more and more states adopt their own legislation, Rhode Island's hearing screening program is looked upon as a model to be replicated. But screening for hearing loss is not an end unto itself—it is a point of departure. The National Institutes of Health Consensus Statement (March, 1993) was explicit in its position that intervention and management services are critical and must be in place when screening programs are established. In looking to Rhode Island's success, one must also look to an entire system where numerous elements—agencies, professionals, physicians, administrators, and most critically families—have worked to create a synergism with subsequent positive outcomes far greater than anyone could accomplish alone. This system assists families and infants at the time of the newborn screening, and continues providing services until the family and child have negotiated the critical first year and the transition into a preschool setting at age three years.

The commitment to hearing screening necessitates a commitment to the development of a total system of care for all families and children with hearing loss, requiring careful analysis and thoughtful, ongoing, responsive change. In

Rhode Island, the system that had been in place for years and that had met the needs of toddlers and preschoolers identified as deaf or hard of hearing, needed to be expanded and recalibrated to meet the needs of infants and their families. The process involved assessment and utilization of existing resources and their funding sources; recognition that each part of the system is equally important to the success of the whole; inclusion of each agency of the system in every decision affecting the system; the development of a plan with clear goals shared by all; and the acknowledgment that parents are the most valuable resource. That acknowledgment prompted the realization the we also needed to recalibrate ourselves and the way in which we work with families.

RECALIBRATING THE SYSTEM

Assessing Resources and Defining Needs

Recalibrating an entire system to a new standard (serving *infants* with hearing loss and their families as well as older children) required new operational goals and initiatives. Resources needed to be identified and to undergo a process of self-evaluation to redefine their roles and contributions to service provision in light of newborn hearing screening. The results of that assessment provided the basis for programmatic and effective change.

Existing programs that served families and young children with special needs and that had areas of strength and expertise, were identified as potential partners in follow-up. Some programs fell under the umbrella of the Department of Health, including the Rhode Island Hearing Assessment Program (RIHAP); Kids Net, a tracking system used by other public health programs; and the statewide system of early intervention. Other programs with expertise in young children with hearing loss, such as the Family Guidance Early Intervention Program based at the Rhode Island School for the Deaf, were under the umbrella of the Department of Education. There were also community-based resources such as a newly formed audiological network that functioned independently of the purview of either state agency. Although each was experiencing a variety of challenges as a result of newborn hearing screening, they functioned without coordination or shared vision and purpose.

A comprehensive needs assessment documented the impact the newborn screening program had on individual programs, and also identified specific areas where new partnerships and initiatives were needed. The first challenge each agency unanimously identified was a dramatic increase in the numbers of referrals to their programs. The Family Guidance Program reported enrollment figures of 18 families participating in May, 1993, more than doubling to 50 families by May, 1999 (see Figure 9–1). The increased referral rate presented such overwhelming problems for our small, specialized staff that we immediately realized we were not prepared for the challenges the screening program had created. The needs assessment helped us recognize the importance of collaborating with community resources that offered specialized services and trained staff. These collaborations would enhance the existing program and were an efficient way to meet the challenge of servicing all the new families and their diverse needs. We looked to the Comprehensive System of Personnel Development (CSPD) within

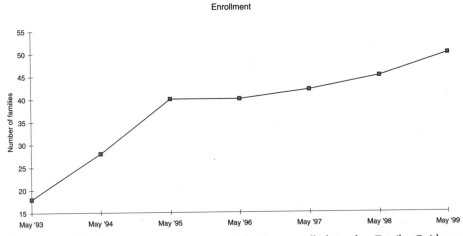

Figure 9-1 Increase in number of families enrolled in the Family Guidance Program after universal newborn hearing screening was legislated in Rhode Island in 1993.

the Department of Health's Early Intervention Program to address these new training needs. The CSPD had already developed a system for training through five working committees that provided opportunities to develop new programming and assessment tools or review existing programs and assessment tools, which could then be adapted for our diverse families.

Programs were straining from the significantly increased demand for their services without an increase in their existing funding sources. Since funding issues can often create barriers to service delivery, we encouraged the Department of Health and the Department of Education to collaborate yet again. The result was a Memorandum of Agreement (MOA) which allows the Department of Education to access Part C funds through the Department of Health to support its early intervention activities. This kind of creative collaboration has made it possible for Rhode Island to successfully serve all of the families identified through RIHAP.

Programs were finding that they needed to respond not only to a change in the number of families requiring early intervention, but to a change in family profiles as well. Of significant interest is the high percentage of children referred who have mild/moderate and unilateral hearing losses (see Figure 9–2). Historically, this population was identified when they entered the school system either during kindergarten or later in the early elementary years. The fact that mild, moderate, and unilateral hearing losses could now be identified in children younger than 6 months of age raised a number of questions regarding amplification, programming, and assessment. Available data were limited regarding appropriate strategies for addressing these families' needs.

Another significant change in family profiles greatly impacted our programs. With the decrease in mortality rates in the neonatal intensive care units (NICU), the number of young children with multiple needs requiring intervention from a range of professionals also had increased. The assessment revealed that these families have significantly different needs and that we were ill-prepared to meet them with the existing staff and resources (see Figure 9–3).

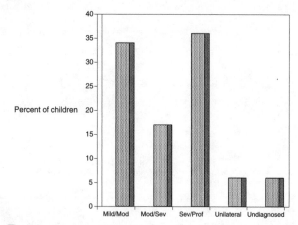

Figure 9-2 Distribution of hearing loss types and degrees.

Implementing a New System of Care: KidsHearing/RI

The needs assessment made it exquisitely clear that no single agency could effectively implement a comprehensive screening and follow-up program. Instead, the following agencies committed to implementing a total system of care which we call KidsHearing/RI.

The Rhode Island Hearing Assessment Program

RIHAP, based at Women and Infants Hospital in Providence, is the program that carries out the legislated mandate for newborn hearing screening on a daily basis, under the direction of the Rhode Island Department of Public Health.

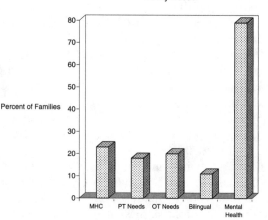

Figure 9-3 Distribution of family needs in addition to those needed for management of hearing loss.

RIHAP manages the process of screening all infants born in any of the state's eight participating hospitals, as well as maintaining an information management system that tracks patients and their screening outcomes. The RIHAP audiologists provide clinical oversight and training to all screening staff, including registered nurses, licensed practical nurses, nurses aides, and technicians. A two-stage screening protocol is utilized, with Stage 1 involving transient evoked otoacoustic emissions (TEOAE) as the primary screening tool. Infants for whom TEOAE cannot be completed or who do not meet the pass criteria enter Stage 2 of the screening process. RIHAP contacts families after discharge and informs them that they should return when their infant is two to four weeks old for screening by automated auditory brainstem response audiometry (AABR). Should pass criteria still not be met, infants are referred for diagnostic audiologic assessment through their local community based sites. RIHAP audiologists play an important role in the first contacts with parents and provide critical audiological information to families, diagnosticians, and service providers.

KIDS NET

KIDS NET is a computerized information management system that tracks children's public health preventive services, with the mission that all Rhode Island children receive comprehensive screening and follow-up for public health preventive services. Some of the services provided by KIDS NET include generating reminders to families when children are due for well-child visits or are overdue for vaccinations or providing information to pediatric providers on-line. In terms of its role in the hearing screening program, KIDS NET Family Outreach Program provides community based outreach and home visits to assist RIHAP in locating or contacting a family in need of RIHAP services or medical intervention. KIDS NET also makes RIHAP hearing screening results and audiological recommendations available electronically to pediatric care providers for babies born on or after January 1, 1997.

Audiology Network

Universal newborn hearing screening precipitated an acute need for quality follow-up services by competent pediatric audiologists. Each self-identified member of this network of certified audiologists, whether employed in private practice, clinic, or hospital-based facility, made a commitment to enhance and improve pediatric audiology in Rhode Island. Members look to protocols based on ASHA guidelines for diagnosis of hearing loss in infants, fitting of amplification for infants, and appropriate audiological follow-up for infants and toddlers. This network is a diagnostic and follow-up resource for families and professionals.

Early Intervention

The Early Intervention Program with its five regional centers promotes the development of infants and toddlers with developmental challenges, and serves eligible children from birth to age three years and their families. Early Intervention helps to identify families' needs and appropriate services through the development of an Individual Family Service Plan (IFSP), based on evaluation recommendations. Those services are then required to be delivered in a family-centered approach. The strongest component of the early intervention program is the important role the parents play in the development of the IFSP and the delivery of services to their child.

Family Guidance Program

The Family Guidance Program based at the Rhode Island School for the Deaf is an early intervention program exclusively for families who have children with hearing loss. Its professional staff (teachers of the deaf, educational audiologists, speech-language pathologists, psychologists, counselors, and visual communication instructors) has expertise in early childhood deafness and hearing loss. It provides all families the support, guidance, and information to empower them with the knowledge and skills needed for making decisions and advocating for their young child. Initial referrals to Family Guidance come from RIHAP and the Department of Health at the time an infant is referred from newborn hearing screening. The staff works collaboratively with the family and the Early Intervention Center serving the family's community, to set goals and identify services that are appropriate to the family and child's needs. The Family Guidance staff provides both center and home-based services for parent support and to help facilitate early communication and language development. Families may be assisted in the process of obtaining appropriate amplification and technology, locating knowledgeable speech-language pathologists, and arranging for further evaluations when warranted. Other available services provided by the Family Guidance Program include: family/parent support groups; parent-to-parent networking; parent-child communication training; guidance in understanding the many and diverse facets of deafness; audiological assessment and management; auditory training; family sign language classes; deaf mentoring; toddler groups, and extended day and daycare programs.

Rhode Island Hearing Center

While many states look to Rhode Island for guidance in creating new screening programs, the fact that the state has a longstanding history of screening its children is overlooked. The Rhode Island Hearing Center is a state-funded audiology facility that was established more than 40 years ago with the mandate to screen the hearing of school-age children. Staffed by trained technicians and audiologists, the Center annually screens 65,000 children from school systems statewide. The Center also provides free audiologic follow-up, including diagnostic assessments and hearing aid evaluations. Over the years, the Center has responded to the growing cultural diversity in the state, running hearing and otologic clinics in neighborhood health centers that served many non–English-speaking communities. We are currently exploring the possibility of scheduling an Hispanic clinic day with a native Spanish-speaking audiologist.

Prior to 1993, the annual statewide school hearing screening program (regulated by the Department of Health and administered through the Department of Education) was the initial gateway for identifying hearing loss in what used to be considered young children. That mechanism for hearing screening continues to play an important role in the overall identification process, although there has been a shift in its function since newborn hearing screening was legislated. School screenings are no longer the original point of identification, but serve as a safety net for children who are new to the system, who did not undergo newborn screening, or who have, in fact, acquired late onset hearing loss. Infants who may have passed the newborn screening may still develop hearing loss in early childhood that must be identified. An important issue for the school screening program to resolve in the future is to determine which children they referred for follow-up were initially flagged as being at risk for hearing loss at the time of newborn screening. It is an imposing task to gather, coordinate, cross-reference, and analyze the results, but certainly an important and necessary one.

Partnerships for Follow-Up Services

A mechanism to link each of the existing resources into an integrated system and add the most important component of the system—the parents—was developed. The *Rhode Island Infant Hearing Screening Advisory Committee* was established as part of the RI legal mandate to provide regulatory oversight of the state system of newborn hearing screening and to serve in an advisory capacity to the Rhode Island Director of Health. Members of the committee represent audiology, pediatrics, insurance, special education, hospital neonatal nurseries, the Deaf community, and the Rhode Island Department of Health. An important function of this committee is to provide professional training regarding newborn screening through an annual conference. The RIHAP Symposium has become a well-recognized and respected continuing education opportunity for practitioners, with leading experts presenting papers on current trends and research.

The *Rhode Island Infant Hearing Screening Follow-Up Committee* functions as a working committee that addresses the practical issues facing parents and professionals vis a vis newborn identification. It was developed to identify and address gaps in services and access barriers for families and professionals; facilitate the process of obtaining funding for amplification; develop protocols in the referral process; develop legislation to facilitate changes in the system; coordinate tracking infants; and to provide educational material to the public. Composed of 25 members, a wide array of professionals, families, agencies, and advocacy groups are represented, including RIHAP, pediatricians, the Department of Health Early Intervention Program, audiologists, speech therapists, mental health professionals, the Deaf community, Alexander Graham Bell Association, Family Outreach, the Department of Education, and most important, parents.

One example of the work that the Follow-Up Committee has recently completed is their monthly quality assurance study. This study group involved early interventionists, audiologists, parents, and educators in a chart review. Quarterly, RIHAP identifies those families who should have entered the early intervention system. This list is electronically checked by the early intervention database. The study group visits each regional early intervention center and reviews the family's record. This process has provided the members with an opportunity to review records documenting several families' journeys from screening to Early Intervention. They were able to review the initial evaluations, the resulting recommendations, and the subsequent Individualized Family Service Plan (IFSP) goals. The members were able to identify any gaps in the process and make recommendations to eliminate those gaps. This process provided many opportunities to ensure that appropriate services were accessible for each family. This Q&A study group has taken its work a step further by making recommendations to effect slight changes so that similar gaps do not occur in the future.

Although these two committees function independently, they both represented a similar theme. Our efforts focus on unifying previously factional organizations by helping them identify their common goal—to develop and implement a quality system for early hearing detection, diagnosis, and intervention that is based on a family-centered approach and adheres to a continuous quality improvement plan. With the leadership of the Department of Education, a Strategic Planning Seminar was held over a two-year period. The Strategic Planning team's members included representatives from the Department of Health Early Intervention Program, the Department of Education, teaching and administrative staff from the Rhode Island School for the Deaf, special education directors from several local communities, the Deaf community, Alexander Graham Bell Association, parents, audiologists, the Rhode Island Hearing Assessment Program, and legal advocates. This committee's goal was to determine the mission, beliefs, and action plans necessary to accomplish our goals in a five-year plan (see Appendix 6–A).

First Connections Resource and Training Project for Newborn Hearing Screening

Funded through a federal grant, First Connections works to ensure that the system of newborn screening and follow-up is cohesive, family centered, and family responsive through continuing educational and training opportunities for the wide range of professionals involved in the process. Families have frequently expressed their stress and anxiety when the diagnosis of hearing loss is first made; audiologic findings and recommendations are inconclusive, contradictory, or inconsistent; specialized speech-language-hearing services are difficult to obtain; and/or their pediatrician or primary care physician is uninformed about hearing loss and the available community resources. Furthermore, members of the "team" rarely have sufficient counseling skills or confidence to address parents' feelings. To address these concerns identified by parents, workshops and seminars about counseling, best practice standards for diagnostic and follow-up audiologic services, critical milestones in early communication and language development, and the role of the physician occur throughout the year.

First Connections has adopted the Joint Committee on Infant Hearing 2000 Postition Statement and the characteristics of the medical home as a framework for refining Rhode Island's Early Hearing Detection and Intervention system. By assuring that services throughout the process are available and comprehensive, coordinated, family centered, compassionate, and culturally competent, the quality of services to families and young children with hearing loss are sure to improve.

RECALIBRATING OURSELVES

Experienced staff members of the Family Guidance Early Intervention Program, along with professionals from the statewide early intervention system, became very aware of a dramatic difference in relationships and work with families whose infants' hearing loss had been identified through newborn screening. It took months of meetings for us to process and define what had changed and how we needed to change in response. In the past, families had time to draw their own conclusions about their child's hearing loss and to recognize the need for intervention. They knew either intuitively or as a result of diagnostic evaluations. Families with toddlers had observed absent or inconsistent auditory responses. They knew their child had communication, speech, and language delays. Many parents had spent months advocating for an audiologic assessment, despite pediatricians who had advised against it or friends and families who saw "nothing wrong." When families were finally referred to the Family Guidance Program, they were relieved to be supported and believed, and they were ready to "go to work." In their own private way, parents had already begun the process of coming to terms with emotions stemming from even the *possibility* their child had a significant hearing loss. The children were older and ready to participate in child-centered, formal intervention. The urgency to establish appropriate programs and strategies so children could acquire language was shared by parents and professionals alike. We were the families' allies and we knew exactly what to do. This is not to say that these families did not experience difficulties that were, at times, overwhelming. Each family experienced the roller coaster ride toward acceptance of their child's deafness, and most moved from one stage to the next just as Kubler-Ross (1969) and Luterman (1979) describe in the literature.

Neonatal hearing screening has created a paradigm shift in the identification process from one that was parent-driven to one that is system-driven (Luterman & Kurtzer-White, 1999). As a result, the dynamic between interventionist and family has changed. Families now enter the program in the initial, acute stages of their grief and are upset over the diagnosis. It is hard for them to believe that anything could possibly be wrong with this sleeping infant and that their lives now involve hearing aids, speech therapy, appointments, and a cadre of professionals knocking on their door. Luterman (1979) has described how parents need to work through the emotions that arise from their sense of loss of the idealized child of their dreams and hopes. Parents become angry at the violation of their expectations, especially when they discover there is no cure for hearing loss. Parents may feel overwhelmed and inadequate to deal with this life change. Furthermore, the identification of hearing loss arises from an external locus: clinicians and medical institutions rather than the families themselves. The diagnosis is being made before parents ever have time to become suspicious. Families now are the recipients of information, rather than proactive seekers of a diagnosis. Instead of the sense of relief or validation parents previously demonstrated at the time of diagnosis, we see a heightened level of anxiety during this time. Although newborn hearing screening is valuable and is the catalyst for early identification of hearing loss in the state, it seems to have the unfortunate side effect of creating a different parental response.

Anyone involved with families of newly identified babies must be prepared to deal with parents' grief. We, too, then must undergo a shift in our own paradigms for providing early intervention. The content-based counseling approaches used in the past to provide information to families is misguided in the earliest stages of diagnosis. Parents are not yet ready for the confusing and often conflicting information endemic to hearing loss and deafness, and professionals may unintentionally add to the parents' stress by providing too much too soon. Luterman (1979) writes, "Information overload can be very harmful because the increased confusion leads to increased feelings of inadequacy and anxiety, all of which tend to reduce self esteem" (p. 61).

Instead, we need to listen to the emotional undertones of what parents are asking or telling us in the early stages of diagnosis, and respond in ways that respect their sadness or pain. For hearing parents' (the majority of children with hearing loss are born to hearing parents), the diagnosis of their baby's hearing loss is a highly emotionally charged event. Our experience is that all parents go through the same grieving process, regardless of the severity of their child's hearing loss. The parents whose child has a mild to moderate hearing loss needs the same emotional supports as the parents whose child has a more severe hearing loss. Speech, hearing parents' intuitive and instinctive means for transmitting their values, culture, emotions, and traditions, suddenly comes to a highly conscious level because of fears that parents and child will not be able to "just talk" to each other. Parents have asked us: "How will I sing Happy Birthday to him?" or "How will she know it's me when I call?" The issues of being able to fully communicate with their child can become enmeshed in their own sense of sufficiency as parents.

We know that the emotional availability of parents is key in helping young children acquire language. We also know that parental belief that baby and adult can and do communicate is critical. Our earliest intervention, then, is our partnerships with parents and placing the parent-child connection at the very center of everything we do. Everything else—hearing aids, technology, speech therapy, sign language—radiates from and to that center. The primacy of the parent-child connection transcends all issues of methodology and technology and is the focus of our work in early intervention (Kurtzer-White, 1999).

Outcome data for successful children transitioning out of the Family Guidance Program point to successful, strong connections between parent and child as the primary contributing factor to the child's progress, not socioeconomic status, modality of communication, or severity of hearing loss. We define a successful connection as being characterized by a reciprocal relationship; parent and child's ability to read and respond to each other's signals and communication; investment in repairing or modifying communication when not understood; an appropriate language model being provided by the parent; and the parent's ability to stay in the moment with their child and to follow his/her communicative lead.

The foundation of our program then is based on helping families to become comfortable with their baby and to help the parents arrive at a style of interaction that is effective and mutually enjoyable for both parent and child. As communication between parent and baby develops and families come to terms with their feelings around the hearing loss, parents can recognize themselves as good and competent parents. There are no intervention techniques more powerful than those that serve to build parental self-esteem (Luterman, 1979). This can be challenging, particularly when families sense the need to "do something" (i.e., fix it) and interventionists focus on the child's deficits. We have seen that this sometimes results in a hyperfocus on technology and concern with obtaining as much speech therapy services as possible for the infant. Programmable hearing aids, FM units, and cochlear implants, while designed to enhance communication can at times detract from parent-child interaction. Earmolds that don't fit, hearing aids that are constantly pulled out and become the source of power struggles, concern that there are new, better and very expensive devices available, and the audiologist's admonition that the child must be amplified during all waking hours can add to a parent's stress. Anxiety over a baby's speech production and focus on inventorying specific speech sounds can also distract from the relationship. Research indicates that the meaning, intent, and success of a baby's communication are more critical in the very early stages of development than its spoken form; however, this can be a difficult concept to successfully convey to parents.

If parent-child connection is our focus, we need to constantly ask ourselves how we can strengthen our partnerships with parents to that end. We looked to anecdotal data we had been collecting on parental responses to a survey on accepting their child's hearing loss. Our results were consonant with those previously published: parents wanted to work with and learn from professionals who are nurturing, who provide unbiased information, and are committed to the family. The results led us to consciously shift from child centeredness to truly family-centered models and realize that our own communication with families has enormous impact. We support families by pointing out all that their babies can do. A reach, a point, or vocalization are important for parents to notice and respond to. And when parents engage in ways that are naturally successful, we also acknowledge the primacy of their contribution to the child's development. We are not in a position to pass judgment, but to meet parents where they are emotionally and to support them as they move through a process toward acceptance and decision making. We understand when parents have a hard time putting hearing aids on their child, just as we understand that families need to often get several opinions from audiologists or other experts. And as difficult as it can be at times, we work to be understanding when parents are angry with us for not having all the answers they want, or when advanced technology fails to fulfill the unspoken promise of helping their child to hear and talk.

The issue of unbiased information is somewhat more complex. When we are truly honest, we recognize that we are biased—everyone is. As experienced educators of the deaf, pediatric audiologists, and language specialists, we believe that our methods are founded in sound theoretical constructs and can result in positive outcomes. We must be honest and open with parents about the views we hold, but never dogmatic. We encourage families to meet other families and professionals with differing biases so that they have a fuller perspective of the many choices available to them. We recognize that this is extraordinarily difficult for families, particularly around the issues of modality. But we also know that families will ultimately make their own best decisions in time when they are well informed and have been able to process the information.

SUMMARY

A comprehensive hearing screening program involves not only detection of hearing loss in infants but a responsive system of follow-up and care for all families whose children are identified with hearing loss. Rhode Island was compelled to recalibrate its existing system because of the significant impact newborn screening had on various programs throughout the state and the realization that the status quo was inadequate. Funding allocations remained limited, forcing careful analysis of available resources and creative solutions to the many issues resulting from newborn screening. Through the enormous efforts of professionals, administrators, parents, the Department of Education, and the Department of Health, a blueprint for a continuum of care has been drawn based on:

- the development of a plan with clear goals shared by all;
- assessment and utilization of existing resources and their funding sources;
- recognition that each part of the system is equally important to the success of the whole;
- inclusion of each agency of the system in every decision affecting the system;
- and the acknowledgment that parents are our most valuable resource.

Universal newborn hearing screening also compelled professionals to recalibrate their programs and the ways in which they worked with families of infants. The profiles and needs of families were seen as different, and the need to shift from child-centered approaches of intervention to those that are truly family centered became imperative. Contributing variables to a child's and families' success included the recognition that:

- There are no intervention techniques more powerful than those that serve to build parental self-esteem (Luterman, 1999).
- The emotional and psychological impact that the diagnosis of hearing loss in infancy has on parents/caretakers must be acknowledged, and parental feelings and behaviors resulting from grief and a sense of loss must be addressed.
- The initial task for parents is to arrive at a style of interaction that is effective and enjoyable where parent and child respond to and influence each other's behaviors.
- Through successful communication, parents and children gain confidence and self-esteem.

Since Rhode Island expanded its hearing screening to include universal newborn screening in 1993, we have found that working with families in the very earliest stages of diagnosis requires time to process and evaluate our own responses and communication with parents. We needed to shift from the content/informational counseling of the past to listening to and validating parents' emotions. We needed to recognize our own biases and to respond honestly to parents' questions and to guide them through a field that is marked by bias. We needed to suspend judgment of what parents should do, with the recognition that each family moves forward at their own pace. We have learned that if parental response is greeted with matching support from the professionals they meet during the first six months to one year following the diagnosis, their anxiety levels should be reduced so that they can become competent, skilled advocates for their child.

ACKNOWLEDGMENTS

The authors gratefully acknowledge colleagues throughout Rhode Island who have committed their time, expertise, and insight to improving services to families and children with hearing loss: Peter Blackwell, Ph.D., Principal of the Rhode Island School for the Deaf; Ron Caldarone, LICSW, Chief of Office of Special Health Care Needs, Rhode Island Department of Health; Ruth H. Schennum, Ph.D., Director of Operations/Early Intervention Program, Rhode Island Department of Health; and Deborah Topol, Language Specialist of the Rhode Island School for the Deaf. Supported in part by PROJECT 1 HGI MC 00009 from the Maternal and Child Health Program (title V, Social Security Act), Health Resources and Service Administration, Department of Health and Human Services.

APPENDIX 9-A

Deciding the Future for Our Children Who Are Deaf or Have Hearing Loss

This document reports the consensus decisions of a broad community of Rhode Island parents, professionals, and citizens devoted to the education of all children from birth to age 21 with hearing loss.

Mission

- proposed as the mission of Rhode Island's statewide system of services impacting all children with hearing loss.

Our mission is to ensure that every child who is deaf or has a hearing loss will become an independent, contributing citizen by harnessing the talents of informed families, competent professionals, and the linguistically and culturally diverse Deaf and hearing communities, to provide fully accessible and appropriate environments to meet the unique educational, social, linguistic, and communication needs of every child.

Beliefs

- proposed as our system's fundamental convictions, values, and character.

We believe that a community with shared beliefs and aspirations that is based on respect and equal opportunity, will thrive and prosper.

We believe that, for a community of participants to have confidence in any process, there must be a shared perspective of integrity in terms of truthfulness and goodwill.

We believe that when diversity among people is experienced and valued, the lives of all are enriched.

We believe that all individuals deserve the opportunity to develop the skills essential to becoming lifelong learners.

We believe that when the community provides opportunities for individuals to develop their talents, and when individuals in turn use their talents in responsible and productive ways, the lives of self and others are enriched.

Strategies

- proposed as desired accomplishments within our statewide system of services.

All children and their families will receive the full spectrum of accurate information and support services to meet their individual needs in a timely fashion.

All families will be encouraged and supported to become active participants in the educational decisions related to their child who has a hearing loss.

The system will ensure that professionals and paraprofessionals working with deaf and hard-of-hearing children and their families will receive ongoing professional development and support, including information about best educational practices.

In order to increase understanding and respect for individual perspectives, all people will become aware of Deaf and hearing issues related to learning, living, and working together in partnership.

We will create an ongoing process to facilitate coordination among agencies, organizations, and the community, and to continuously build partnerships among Deaf, hard of hearing, and hearing people.

Objectives

• proposed as the desired results for children.

By age three, all children who are deaf or have a hearing loss will develop the social, communicative, learning, and language skills that are a necessary foundation for school readiness.

All students who are deaf or have a hearing loss will develop the learning and communication strategies, language competence, and reading and writing skills necessary to meet national and state standards of achievement in language arts, math, science, and social studies.

All children who are deaf or have a hearing loss will graduate from high school. Within one year of graduation, all graduates who are deaf or have a hearing loss will be participating in an educational experience, be gainfully employed, or be pursuing other personal goals.

REFERENCES

American Speech-Language-Hearing Association. (1979). Guidelines for acoustic immittance screening of middle ear function. *ASHA*, 283–288.

American Speech-Language-Hearing Association. (1990). Guidelines for screening for hearing impairments and middle-ear disorders. *ASHA*, 32(Suppl. 2), 17–24.

American Speech-Language-Hearing Association. (1997). *Guidelines for audiologic screening*. Rockville, MD.

Bess, F., et al. (1978). Use of acoustic impedance measurement in screening for middle ear disease in children. *Annals of Otology, Rhinology and Laryngology, 87*(2), 3–5.

Bluestone, C., et al. (1986). Controversies in screening for middle ear disease and hearing loss in children. *Pediatrics, 77*(1), 57–71.

Calderone, R. (1998). Diagnosis to intervention: infrastructure, funding, quality assurance. Paper presented at the Centers for Disease Control and Prevention Workshop on Early Hearing Detection and Identification. Atlanta, GA.

Johnson, M. J. (1998). Local issues related to intervention for deaf and hearing-impaired children. Paper presented at the Centers for Disease Control and Prevention Workshop on Early Hearing Detection and Identification. Atlanta, GA.

Kubler-Ross, E. (1969). *On death and dying*. New York: Macmillan, 1969.

Kurtzer-White, E. (1999). *The young deaf child*. Baltimore, MD: York Press.

Luterman, D. (1979). *Counseling parents of hearing impaired children*. Boston, MA: Little, Brown and Company.

Luterman, D. (1996). *Persons with communication disorders and their families*. Austin, TX: Pro Ed.

Luterman, D., & Kurtzer-White, E. (1999). Identifying hearing loss: Parents' needs. *American Journal of Audiology, 8*, 13–18.

National Institute on Deafness and Other Communication Disorders (1993, March 1–3). *National Institutes of Health Consensus Statement: Early identification of hearing impairment in infants and young children*. Bethesda, MD.

Shontz, F. (1967). Reactions to crisis. *Volta Review, 69*.

Epilogue:
Communicating with Families

Jackson Roush

When told that their child may have a hearing loss or middle ear disorder, most parents are understandably concerned. These conditions are well known to health care providers, but to many parents they are unfamiliar and disturbing. Furthermore, unlike most routine health screening procedures there may be a delay of days or even weeks before follow-up is completed. Thus, the information provided and how it is conveyed are issues of major importance. Even when skillfully communicated, however, many parents will worry until the question is resolved. Consequently, there is a serious professional obligation to provide clear and accurate information to families along with a timely and appropriate plan for follow-up. As noted throughout this text, the specifics of follow-up will vary based on the nature of the referral, family preferences, available resources, financial arrangements, and program design. But the desired outcome is the same: a clear and forthright explanation of the screening results and the specific steps needed for follow-up.

INITIAL REFERRAL BASED ON HEARING SCREENING

It is important to remember that many young children referred for follow-up testing, especially those seen in conjunction with a universal newborn infant hearing-screening program, will eventually be found to have normal hearing. This fact needs to be communicated to parents when screening results are reported, but reassurance must be balanced with sufficient emphasis on the importance of returning for follow-up. In general, it is preferable to avoid the terms "fail" or "failure" when reporting a screening outcome, opting instead for terminology such as "did not pass," or simply "refer." A father recently shared his reaction to being told that his newborn son had failed a hearing screening: "He wasn't even a day old and had already failed something!" No matter how routine the testing and reporting become, those involved with the screening program need to remember that the family is receiving this information for the first time. Moreover, the news comes at a time when family members, especially the mother, may be physically and emotionally exhausted. Carefully worded written materials, presented at a level (and in a language) appropriate for families, are a necessary supplement to verbal reporting of screening outcomes. When referral is needed many programs supplement this communication with a follow-up letter, restating the results and referral procedures and providing a phone number to call if they have questions.

WHEN SHOULD FAMILIES BE INFORMED?

There are differences of opinion regarding the optimal time to inform families of the newborn hearing screening outcome. While most programs inform parents prior to hospital discharge, some choose to wait two or three weeks. This waiting period is intended to allow families time to recover from the delivery and to enjoy the initial bonding period without the anxiety of a possible hearing loss. But waiting increases the chances of babies being lost to follow-up. Communication from hospital to home may be difficult, especially when there are linguistic or cultural barriers. Furthermore, some parents are annoyed if not informed immediately of any concerns regarding their child's hearing. Still, the practical advantages of informing families prior to discharge are justifiable only if communication is handled skillfully and accurately.

WHO INFORMS THE FAMILY?

Programs vary with regard to who delivers the information. In a well-baby or high-risk nursery, screening results are often reported by a nurse, although some programs choose to have an audiologist report the outcome when referral is needed. In a preschool or school-age setting the information is conveyed through written communication since screening is usually performed when parents are not present. Regardless of who is assigned this responsibility, screening personnel must appreciate the importance of their role and the impact of the news they deliver. Unfortunately, parent surveys indicate that communication with families is sometimes handled with little attention to how the information is imparted. For every program, the decision of who informs families and how the information is delivered is of utmost importance. Obviously, the information must be delivered in the family's native language, at a level they can easily comprehend. In addition to providing an interpretation of the screening results, the person assigned to this role must be prepared to answer questions and/or refer the family to an audiologist for further information.

WHEN PERMANENT HEARING LOSS IS SUSPECTED

When a sensorineural hearing loss appears likely, careful communication with families is imperative. The literature is replete with testimonials from parents describing the cold, technical manner in which they were informed of their child's hearing loss. While it is presumed that most practitioners are skilled in dealing with parents at this critical early stage, the importance of delivering information clearly and accurately, with sensitivity to the emotional impact of this news, cannot be overstated. Parents typically have many questions regarding the nature of their child's hearing loss and how they should proceed with intervention. For nearly all parents, this is a stressful and uncertain period with profound implications for the entire family. The direct involvement of an audiologist at this stage is essential. If hearing loss is confirmed by audiologic assessment, the family will be referred to an otolaryngologist for medical examination and to a public agency to explore intervention options. Federal and state laws require that referral be made to a public agency within two days of identification and that a multidisciplinary assessment be scheduled within 45 days to determine eligibility for special services. Children with permanent bilateral hearing loss will almost always qualify for intervention services. Documentation in the form of an Individualized Family Service Plan (for infants and toddlers) or an Individualized Education Plan (for preschool and school-aged children) is required by law in all fifty states.

WHEN OTITIS MEDIA IS SUSPECTED

Otitis media, although less serious than permanent hearing loss, also requires skillful communication with families. When informing parents of a middle ear disorder and the need for medical follow-up it is important to remember that although OME is a transient condition that often resolves without treatment, there can sometimes be serious medical complications. Furthermore, chronic or recurrent OME may effect speech, language, learning, and socialization, especially in children who are already experiencing developmental delays. Thus, reassurance must be balanced with sufficient urgency to encourage timely follow-up.

CONFIDENTIALITY AND INFORMED CONSENT

It was noted throughout this text that parental permission must be obtained prior to conducting hearing and middle ear screening procedures. In many settings, consent is obtained as part of an institutional enrollment process or admission procedure. Failure to obtain informed consent is not only unprofessional but personnel responsible for the screening program and their institutions are open to negative public relations and possible legal action. Parents have a right to be informed of any proposed screening procedures and their purpose. In addition to informed consent, strict confidentiality must be assured. Discussion of screening outcomes or distribution of results is not permitted without their knowledge and consent, and mechanisms used to transmit screening results must be in secure data formats. Most screening programs have institutional guidelines for informed consent, protection of confidentiality, and secure distribution of test results. If guidelines do not exist, they must be implemented according to institutional protocols as well as state and federal laws. Screening personnel must be familiar with these policies and maintain their full compliance at all times.

CONCLUSIONS

Every child, regardless of age or developmental status, is unique and extraordinary to his or her family. The arrival of a newborn infant evokes powerful emotions. For most families the birth of a child is among the most memorable and distinctive events ever to be experienced. Professionals whose responsibilities necessitate an intrusion at this time must fully appreciate the impact of everything they do and say. This is also true when dealing with parents of older children. Competent and effective communication with families is every bit as essential to a screening program as the technical and administrative components. A comprehensive plan that gives sufficient attention to the interpersonal as well as technical elements will succeed in accomplishing the most important goal of any screening program: timely and appropriate identification, referral and follow-up for every child.

Glossary

Acoustic admittance battery—series of tests designed to measure the flow of acoustic energy through the middle ear system.

Acoustic millimhos (mmho)—unit of measure for acoustic admittance.

Acoustic reflex (AR)—reflexive contraction of the stapedius muscle in response to loud sound.

Acute—of sudden onset and short duration.

Acute purulent otitis media—acute inflammation of the middle ear with infection.

Air conduction pathway—the transmission of sound through the outer and middle ear to the cochlea.

Air conduction threshold—the hearing threshold for a pure tone stimulus delivered from an earphone or insert receiver.

American Academy of Audiology (AAA)—a national professional association of audiologists.

American Speech-Language-Hearing Association (ASHA)—a national professional association of audiologists, speech-language pathologists, and speech, hearing, and language scientists.

Audiogram—graphic representation of hearing thresholds plotted as a function of stimulus frequency.

Audiologist—a healthcare professional whose practices include prevention, evaluation, and rehabilitation of hearing loss and related communication disorders.

Auditory brainstem response—neurological responses produced by the eighth nerve and brainstem in response to an auditory stimulus.

Auditory neuropathy—a term used to describe a pattern of symptoms in which behavioral or physiologic measures suggest significant hearing loss, yet measures of cochlear function, specifically outer hair cell function, appear normal.

Basilar membrane—a membrane of the cochlea that forms a boundary between the scala vestibuli and scala tympani; supports the organ of Corti.

Behavioral hearing tests—assessment procedures involving observable responses to auditory stimuli.

Bilateral hearing loss—a reduction of hearing sensitivity in both ears.

Bone conduction—transmission of sound to the cochlea by vibration of the skull and surrounding tissue.

Bone conduction threshold—the threshold of hearing sensitivity to pure tone stimuli delivered via a bone conduction oscillator.

Calibration—the adjustment of an instrument's output to a known standard.

Central auditory processing disorder (CAPD)—a functional disorder of auditory processing resulting from diseases, trauma, or abnormal development of the central auditory nervous system.

Cerumen—secreted substance of the ceruminous glands in the ear canal, commonly referred to as "ear wax."

Cochlea—auditory portion of the inner ear, consisting of fluid-filled membranous channels.

Cochlear implant—a device consisting of an electrode array surgically implanted in the cochlea; delivers electrical signals to the auditory nerve from an external processor enabling persons with profound hearing loss to perceive sound.

Conductive hearing loss—reduction in hearing sensitivity, despite normal cochlear function, caused by impaired sound transmission through the external ear canal, tympanic membrane, or middle ear ossicles.

Distortion product otoacoustic emissions (DPOAE)—cochlear emissions resulting from simultaneous presentation of two pure tones resulting in a third (distortion) tone.

Ear infection—see acute purulent otitis media.

Endolymph—fluid contained in the scala media of the cochlea.

Equivalent volume—an acoustic immittance measurement that provides an estimate of physical volume.

Etiology—the cause of a disease or condition.

Eustachian tube—passageway leading from the nasopharynx (throat) to the anterior wall of the middle ear; opens during yawning and swallowing to equalize middle ear air pressure.

Frequency—for a sine wave, the number of cycles occurring in 1 second; expressed as Hertz (Hz).

Hair cells—sensory cells of the organ of Corti where nerve endings from the VIIIth nerve terminate.

Hearing level (HL)—the decibel level of sound referenced to the average threshold of sensitivity for young healthy listeners; used on audiograms and audiometers, expressed as dB HL.

Helicotrema—passage at the apical end of the cochlea, connecting the scala tympani and the scala vestibuli.

Incidence—frequency of occurrence, expressed as the number of new cases of a disease or condition in a specified population, over a specified time period, usually one year.

Incus—middle bone of the ossicular chain.

Malleus—largest and most lateral bone of the ossicular chain, attached at one end to the tympanic membrane and on the other to the incus.

Masking noise—sound used by an audiologist to eliminate the participation of one ear while testing the other.

Mastoid process—conical projection of the temporal bone, lying posterior and inferior to the external auditory canal; creates a bony prominence behind and below the auricle.

Membranous labyrinth—fluid-filled channels within the osseous labyrinth of the inner ear, containing the end organ structures for hearing and vestibular function.

Meningitis—a bacterial or viral inflammation of the meninges; can result in significant auditory disorder caused by infection or inflammation of the inner ear or auditory nerve.

Mixed hearing loss—hearing loss with both conductive and sensorineural components.

Nasopharynx—cavity of the nose and pharynx where the eustachian tube opens.

Negative predictive value (NPV)—probability that a disorder is not present when a test is negative.

Noninvasive—a procedure that does not involve penetration of the skin, for example, the use of surface electrodes in auditory brainstem response recording.

Objective test procedure—measurement of hearing sensitivity based on predictions made from physiologic responses to sound, not requiring the active participation of the patient.

Organ of Corti—hearing organ, composed of sensory and supporting cells, located in the cochlear duct on the basilar membrane.

Osseous labyrinth—channels that connect the petrous portion of the temporal bone; contains the membranous labyrinth of the inner ear.

Ossicles—the three small bones of the middle ear (malleus, incus, and stapes) extending from the tympanic membrane through the middle ear cavity to the oval window.

Ossicular chain—collective reference to the three ossicles.

Otalgia—ear pain.

Otic capsule—osseous portion of the cochlea containing the membranous labyrinth of the inner ear.

Otitis externa—infectious or non-infectious conditions resulting in inflammation of the ear canal; may be accompanied by pain, swelling, and otorrhea.

Otitis media (OM)—inflammation of the middle ear.

Otitis media with effusion (OME)—inflammation of the middle ear with an accumulation of fluid in the middle ear cavity.

Otoacoustic emissions (OAE)—low-level sounds emitted by the cochlea, either spontaneously or in response to an auditory stimulus; generated by the outer hair cells of the cochlea.

Otolaryngologist—physician specializing in the diagnosis and treatment of diseases of the ear, nose, and throat, including diseases of related structures of the head and neck.

Otorrhea—discharge from the ear.

Otoscope—an optical device that provides light and magnification for the visual examination of the external auditory canal and tympanic membrane.

Oval window—opening in the labyrinthine wall of the middle ear space leading into the scala vestibuli of the cochlea; point of ossicular attachment for the stapes.

Perilymph—cochlear fluid, found in the scala vestibuli, scala tympani, and spaces within the organ of Corti.

Positive predictive value (PPV)—probability that a disorder is present when a test is positive.

Post-stimulus latency—time interval between the presentation of an acoustic stimulus and initiation of a response.

Predictive value—probability that the result of a given test, positive or negative, is an indicator of the presence or absence of a disorder.

Presbycusis—hearing impairment associated with advancing age.

Prevalence—number of existing cases of a specific disease or condition in a given population at a given time.

Primaries—two pure tones presented as stimuli for the production of a distortion product otoacoustic emission (DPOAE).

Pure tone air conduction audiometry—measurement of hearing thresholds to pure tone stimuli presented through earphones or insert receivers.

Pure tone audiometer—an instrument for presenting pure tone stimuli of selected frequencies at calibrated output levels for hearing screening or for determination of hearing thresholds.

Pure tone bone conduction audiometry—measurement of hearing thresholds to pure tone stimuli presented via a bone vibrator placed on the forehead or mastoid.

Pure tone screening—measurement of hearing sensitivity to pure tone signals at a fixed hearing level, typically 20 dB HL, for pure tone stimuli.

Pure tone threshold audiometry—determination of the lowest level a pure tone stimulus can be detected approximately 50% of the time.

Recessive genetic conditions—inherited condition in which both parents carry an abnormal gene; on average, 25% of offspring are affected.

Reissner's membrane—membrane within the cochlear duct that separates the scala vestibuli and scala media.

Rubella—a viral infection characterized by fever and a transient skin rash resembling measles; may result in abnormalities in the fetus, including sensorineural hearing loss (also known as German measles).

Scala media—middle of three channels of the cochlear duct, bordered by the basilar membrane, Reissner's membrane, and the spiral ligament; contains endolymph and the organ of Corti.

Scala tympani—lower channel of the cochlear duct, separated by the scala media; contains perilymph.

Scala vestibuli—upper channel of the cochlear duct, separated by the scala media; contains perilymph.

Screening—the process of identifying individuals most likely to have a disorder from an asymptomatic population. The screening procedures described in this text are designed to identify children most likely to have a hearing or middle ear disorder so they can be referred for medical and/or audiologic management.

Sensitivity—the ability of a test to identify the disorder it was designed to detect; expressed as the percentage of positive results in individuals known to have the disorder, i.e., the percentage of affected individuals correctly identified.

Sensorineural hearing loss—loss of hearing sensitivity caused by disorders involving the cochlea and/or the auditory nerve.

Serous otitis media—inflammation of the middle ear, with an accumulation of thin, watery (serous) fluid.

Sound level meter—an instrument designed to measure sound pressure level in dB according to an accepted standard.

Sound pressure level (SPL)—magnitude or quantity of sound energy relative to a standard reference pressure.

Specificity—the ability of a test to differentiate a normal condition from the disorder the test was designed to detect; expressed as the percentage of negative results in individuals without the disorder, i.e., the percent of non-effected individuals correctly classified.

Speech-language pathologist—healthcare professional whose practices include evaluation, rehabilitation, and prevention of speech and language disorders.

Stapedius muscle—one of two muscles of the middle ear; the stapedius contracts in response to loud sounds.

Stapes—smallest and most medial bone of the ossicular chain.

Stereocilia—hair-like projections arising from the apical end of the inner and outer hair cells.

Tectorial membrane—gelatinous membrane within the scala media where some of the cilia from the outer hair cells are embedded.

Threshold audiometry—measurement of hearing to determine the lowest sound pressure level at which an acoustic signal can be detected.

Transient evoked otoacoustic emission (TEOAE)—low-level acoustic signal emitted by the cochlea in response to a click or transient auditory stimulus; related to the integrity and function of the outer hair cells of the cochlea.

Tympanic membrane—thin, membranous tissue at the terminal end of the external auditory meatus and forming the major portion of the lateral wall of the middle ear cavity. Its vibrations in response to sound are transferred to the ossicular chain by its connection to the malleus.

Tympanogram—graph of middle ear immittance as a function of air pressure changes created in the ear canal.

Tympanometer—instrument used to assess middle ear function through measurement of the acoustic immittance of the tympanic membrane and middle ear, as air pressure delivered to the ear canal is varied.

Tympanometric width—the width of the pressure peak on a tympanogram, reported as the pressure interval (in daPa) that corresponds with a 50% reduction in static admittance.

Tympanostomy tube—small tube inserted in the tympanic membrane to equalize air pressure in the middle ear.

Unilateral hearing loss—loss of hearing sensitivity in one ear only.

Validity—the extent to which a test measures what it is intended to measure.

AMERICAN
SPEECH-LANGUAGE-
HEARING
ASSOCIATION

ASHA

| HOME | SEARCH SITE | CONTENTS | CONTACT US |

Joint Committee on Infant Hearing

INFANT
HEARING
SCREENING

Background

References

Model Bill

Write to Congress

State Status

Join EdNet and
HealthNet

Year 2000 Position Statement: Principles and Guidelines for Early Hearing Detection and Intervention Programs

The Year 2000 Position Statement and Guidelines were developed by the Joint Committee on Infant Hearing (JCIH). Joint Committee member organizations and their respective representatives who prepared this statement include (in alphabetical order) the American Academy of Audiology (Terese Finitzo, PhD, chair; and Yvonne Sininger, PhD); the American Academy of Otolaryngology—Head and Neck Surgery (Patrick Brookhouser, MD, vice-chair; and Stephen Epstein, MD); the American Academy of Pediatrics (Allen Erenberg, MD; and Nancy Roizen, MD); the American Speech-Language-Hearing Association (Allan O. Diefendorf, PhD; Judith S. Gravel, PhD; and Richard C. Folsom, PhD); the Council on Education of the Deaf whose member organizations include Alexander Graham Bell Association for the Deaf and Hard of Hearing, American Society for Deaf Children, Conference of Educational Administrators of Schools and Programs for the Deaf, Convention of American Instructors of the Deaf, National Association of the Deaf, and Association of College Educators of the Deaf and Hard of Hearing (Patrick Stone, EdD; Joseph J. Innes, PhD; and Donna M. Dickman, PhD); and the Directors of Speech and Hearing Programs in State Health and Welfare Agencies (Lorraine Michel, PhD.; Linda Rose, MCD; and Thomas Mahoney, PhD). Ex officios to the JCIH include Evelyn Cherow, MA (American Speech-Language Hearing Association); Deborah Hayes, PhD (Marion Downs National Center for Infant Hearing); and Liz Osterhus, MA, and Thomas Tonniges, MD (American Academy of Pediatrics).*

Joint Committee member organizations that adopt this statement include (in alphabetical order) the American Academy of Audiology, the American Academy of Pediatrics, the American Speech-Language-Hearing Association (LC 7–2000), the Council on Education of the Deaf (see above individual organizations), and the Directors of Speech and Hearing Programs in State Health and Welfare Agencies.

*Donna Dickman, deceased.

TABLE OF CONTENTS

The Position Statement

References

THE POSITION STATEMENT

The Joint Committee on Infant Hearing (JCIH) endorses early detection of, and intervention for infants with hearing loss (early hearing detection and intervention, EHDI) through integrated, interdisciplinary state and national systems of universal newborn hearing screening, evaluation, and family-centered intervention. The goal of EHDI is to maximize linguistic and communicative competence and literacy development for children who are hard of hearing or deaf. Without appropriate opportunities to learn language, children who are hard of hearing or deaf will fall behind their hearing peers in language, cognition, and social-emotional development. Such delays may result in lower educational and employment levels in adulthood (Gallaudet University Center for Assessment and Demographic Study, 1998). Thus, all infants' hearing should be screened using objective, physiologic measures in order to identify those with congenital or neonatal onset hearing loss. Audiologic evaluation and medical evaluations should be in progress before 3 months of age. Infants with confirmed hearing loss should receive intervention before 6 months of age from health care and education professionals with expertise in hearing loss and deafness in infants and young children. Regardless of prior hearing screening outcomes, all infants who demonstrate risk indicators for delayed onset or progressive hearing loss should receive ongoing audiologic and medical monitoring for 3 years and at appropriate intervals thereafter to ensure prompt identification and intervention (American Speech-Language-Hearing Association, 1997). EHDI systems should guarantee seamless transitions for infants and their families through this process.

Appropriate early intervention programs are family-centered, interdisciplinary, culturally competent, and build on informed choice for families (Baker-Hawkins & Easterbrooks, 1994). To achieve informed decision making, families should have access to professional, educational, and consumer organizations, and they should have opportunities to interact with adults and children who are hard of hearing and deaf (Ogden, 1996; Thompson, 1994). Families should have access to general information on child development and specific information on hearing loss and language development. To achieve accountability, individual community and state, health and educational programs should assume the responsibility for coordinated, ongoing measurement and improvement of EHDI process outcomes.

I. Background

Hearing loss in newborns and infants is not readily detectable by routine clinical procedures (behavioral observation), although parents often report the suspicion of hearing loss, inattention, or erratic response to sound before hearing loss is confirmed (Arehart, Yoshinaga-Itano, Thomson, Gabbard, & Stredler Brown, 1998; Harrison & Roush, 1996; Kile, 1993). The average age of identification in the United States is being reduced with EHDI programs; until very recently, it had been 30 months of age (Harrison & Roush, 1996). Although children who have severe to profound hearing loss or multiple disabilities may be identified before 30 months, children with mild-to-moderate losses often are not identified until school age because of the nature of hearing loss and the resultant inconsistent response to sound (Elssmann, Matkin, & Sabo, 1987). For this reason, the National Institute on Deafness and Other Communication Disorders (of the National Institutes of Health) released a Consensus Statement on Early Identification of Hearing Impairment in Infants and Young Children in 1993. The statement concluded that all infants admitted to the neonatal intensive care unit (NICU) should be screened for hearing loss before hospital discharge and that universal screening should be implemented for all infants within the first 3 months of life (NIDCD, 1993). In its 1994 Position Statement, the JCIH endorsed the goal of universal detection of infants with hearing loss and encouraged continuing research and development to improve methodologies for identification of and intervention for hearing loss (Joint Committee on Infant Hearing, 1994a, 1994b, 1995a, 1995b).

In the ensuing years, considerable data have been reported that support not only the feasibility of universal newborn hearing screening (UNHS) but also the benefits of early intervention for infants with hearing loss (Moeller, in press). Specifically, infants who are hard of hearing and deaf who receive intervention before 6 months of age maintain language development commensurate with their cognitive abilities through the age of 5 years (Yoshinaga-Itano, 1995; Yoshinaga-Itano, Sedey, Coulter, & Mehl, 1998). Numerous investigators have documented the validity, reliability, and effectiveness of early detection of infants who are hard of hearing and deaf through universal newborn hearing screening (Finitzo, Albright, & O'Neal, 1998; Prieve and Stevens, 2000; Spivak, 1998; Spivak et al., 2000; Vohr, Carty, Moore, & Letourneau, 1998; Vohr & Maxon, 1996). Cost-effective screening is being undertaken in individual hospitals and in numerous statewide programs in the United States (Arehart, Yoshinaga-Itano, Thomson, Gabbard, & Stredler Brown, 1998; Finitzo, Albright, & O'Neal, 1998; Mason & Hermann, 1998; Mehl & Thomson, 1998; Vohr, Carty, Moore, & Letourneau, 1998). As of Spring 2000, more than half of the States have enacted legislation supporting universal newborn hearing screening. Working groups convened by the National Institute on Deafness and Other Communication Disorders (NIDCD) in 1997 and 1998 offered recommendations on Acceptable Protocols for Use in State-Wide Universal Newborn Hearing Screening Programs and Characterization of Auditory Performance and Intervention Strategies Following Neonatal Screening (NIDCD, 1997, 1998). Given these findings and empirical evidence to date, the JCIH considers that accepted public health criteria have been met to justify implementation of universal newborn hearing screening (American Academy of Pediatrics, 1999a,b; American Speech-Language-Hearing Association, 1989; Spivak, 1998). The JCIH issues the year 2000 Position Statement, describes principles underlying effective EHDI programs, and provides an accompanying guideline on implementing and maintaining a successful EHDI program.

II. Principles

The Joint Committee on Infant Hearing (JCIH) endorses the development of family-centered, community-based EHDI systems. EHDI systems are comprehensive, coordinated, timely, and available to all infants. The following eight principles provide the foundation for effective EHDI systems. Each of the principles is discussed in the Guideline, which follows the delineation of the principles.

1. All infants have access to hearing screening using a physiologic measure. Newborns who receive routine care have access to hearing screening during their hospital birth admission. Newborns in alternative birthing facilities, including home births, have access to and are referred for screening before 1 month of age. All newborns or infants who require neonatal intensive care receive hearing screening before discharge from the hospital. These components constitute universal newborn hearing screening (UNHS).

2. All infants who do not pass the birth admission screen and any subsequent rescreening begin appropriate audiologic and medical evaluations to confirm the presence of hearing loss before 3 months of age.

3. All infants with confirmed permanent hearing loss receive services before 6 months of age in interdisciplinary intervention programs that recognize and build on strengths, informed choice, traditions, and cultural beliefs of the family.

4. All infants who pass newborn hearing screening but who have risk indicators for other auditory disorders and/or speech and language delay receive ongoing audiologic and medical surveillance and monitoring for communication development. Infants with indicators associated with late-onset, progressive, or fluctuating hearing loss as well as auditory neural conduction disorders and/or brainstem auditory pathway dysfunction should be monitored.

5. Infant and family rights are guaranteed through informed choice, decision-making, and consent.

6. Infant hearing screening and evaluation results are afforded the same protection as all other health care and educational information. As new standards for privacy and confidentiality are proposed, they must balance the needs of society and the rights of the infant and family, without compromising the ability of health and education to provide care (AAP, 1999).

7. Information systems are used to measure and report the effectiveness of EHDI services. Although state registries measure and track screening, evaluation, and intervention outcomes for infants and their families, efforts should be made to honor a family's privacy by removing identifying information wherever possible. Aggregate state and national data may also be used to measure and track the impact of EHDI programs on public health and education while maintaining the confidentiality of individual infant and family information.

8. EHDI programs provide data to monitor quality, demonstrate compliance with legislation and regulations, determine fiscal accountability and cost effectiveness, support reimbursement for services, and mobilize and maintain community support.

III. Guidelines for Early Hearing Detection and Intervention Programs

These Guidelines are developed to supplement the eight JCIH Year 2000 Position Statement Principles and to support the goals of universal access to hearing screening, evaluation, and intervention for newborns and infants embodied in Healthy People 2000 (U.S. Department of Health and Human Services Public Health Service, 1990) and 2010 (U.S. Department of Health and Human Services, 2000). The Guidelines provide current information on the development and implementation of successful EHDI systems.

Hearing screening should identify infants at risk for specifically defined hearing loss that interferes with development. On the basis of investigations of long-term, developmental consequences of hearing loss in infants, current limitations of physiologic screening techniques, availability of effective intervention, and in concert with established principles of health screening (American Academy of Pediatrics, 1999b; Fletcher, Fletcher, & Wagner, 1988; Sackett, Haynes, & Tugwell, 1991), the JCIH defines the targeted hearing loss for UNHS programs as permanent bilateral or unilateral, sensory or conductive hearing loss, averaging 30 to 40 dB or more in the frequency region important for speech recognition (approximately 500 through 4000 Hz). The JCIH recommends that all infants with the targeted hearing loss be identified so that appropriate intervention and monitoring may be initiated.

Hearing loss as defined above has effects on communication, cognition, behavior, social-emotional development, and academic outcomes and later vocational opportunities (Karchmer & Allen, 1999). These effects have been well documented by large-scale research investigations in children with (a) mild-to-profound bilateral hearing loss (Bess & McConnell, 1981; Blair, Peterson, & Vieweg, 1985; Carney & Moeller, 1998; Davis, Elfenbein, Schum, & Bentler, 1986; Davis, Shepard, Stelmachowicz, & Gorga, 1981; Karchmer & Allen, 1999), (b) moderate-to-profound unilateral sensorineural hearing loss (Bess & Tharpe, 1984, 1986; Oyler, Oyler, & Matkin, 1988), and (c) minimal flat or sloping sensory hearing loss (Bess, Dodd-Murphy, & Parker, 1998). The incidence and/or prevalence of these types of hearing loss have also been described (Bess, Dodd-Murphy, & Parker, 1998; Dalzell et al., 2000; Finitzo, Albright, & O'Neal, 1998; Mehl & Thomson, 1998). For children with mild-to-profound bilateral sensory hearing loss, effective habilitation strategies including use of personal amplification, language development programs, and speech training have been described (Goldberg & Flexer, 1993; Stelmacho-wicz, 1999; Yoshinaga-Itano, Sedey, Coulter, & Mehl, 1998).

Depending on the screening technology selected, infants with hearing loss less than 30 dB HL or with hearing loss related to auditory neuropathy or neural conduction disorders may not be detected in a universal newborn hearing screening program. Although the JCIH recognizes that these disorders may result in developmental delay, limitations of some currently recommended screening technologies preclude cost-effective detection of these disorders. All infants, regardless of newborn hearing screening outcome, should receive ongoing monitoring for development of age-appropriate auditory behaviors and communication skills. Any infant who demonstrates delayed auditory and/or communication skills development should receive audiologic evaluation to rule out hearing loss.

The JCIH supports applying the concepts of continual process or quality improvement to each component of EHDI programs to achieve desired outcomes. The JCIH recommends that systems be designed to achieve quality outcomes for infants and their families and for hospital, state, and national programs. Specifically, at each step in the process of care, performance measures should be undertaken to examine whether the system conforms to accepted standards of quality (Finitzo, 1999; Tharpe & Clayton, 1997). This guideline outlines the benchmarks and associated quality indicators that serve to monitor compliance and outcomes at each step in the EHDI process.

Benchmarks are quantifiable goals or targets by which an EHDI program may be monitored and evaluated. Benchmarks are used to evaluate progress and to point to needed next steps in achieving and maintaining a quality EHDI program (O'Donnell & Galinsky, 1998). Because EHDI programs are relatively new, the JCIH has included examples of established benchmarks that are based on existing data and suggested benchmarks in areas where published data are not currently available. Quality indicators reflect a result in relation to a stated benchmark. Quality indicators should be monitored using well-established practices of statistical process control to determine program consistency and stability (Wheeler & Chambers, 1986). If the quality indicators demonstrate that a program is not meeting the stated benchmark, sources of variability should be identified and corrected to improve the process (Tharpe & Clayton, 1997). It is prudent for hospitals and state programs to establish a periodic review process to evaluate benchmarks as more data on EHDI outcomes become available and to examine how program quality indicators are conforming to established benchmarks.

A. Roles and Responsibilities

1. Institutions and Agencies. A variety of public and private institutions and agencies may assume responsibility for specific components (e.g., screening, evaluation, intervention) of a comprehensive EHDI program and the training required for EHDI success. State and local agencies that are involved in components of an EHDI program should work collaboratively to define their roles, responsibilities, and accountability. These roles and responsibilities may differ from state to state; however, it is strongly recommended that each state identify a lead coordinating agency with oversight responsibility for EHDI. The lead coordinating agency should convene an advisory committee consisting of professionals, families with children who are hard of hearing or deaf, members of the hard of hearing and Deaf communities, and other interested community leaders to provide guidance on the development, coordination, funding, and quality evaluation of community-based EHDI programs (ASHA, AAA, & AG Bell, 1997; Model Universal Newborn/Infant Hearing Screening, Tracking, and Intervention Bill). The lead coordinating agency in each state should be responsible for identifying the public and private funding sources available to support development, implementation, and coordination of EHDI systems. Funding sources may vary from year to year. Currently, federal sources of systems support include Title V block grants to states for maternal and child health care services, Title XIX (Medicaid) federal and state funds for eligible children, and competitive U.S. Department of Education demonstration and research grants. The National Institute on Deafness and Other Communication Disorders provides grants for research related to early identification and intervention for children who are hard of hearing and deaf. Sources of reimbursement for services to individual children will vary from state to state and may include private medical insurance coverage.

2. Families and Professionals. The success of EHDI programs depends on professionals working in partnership with families as a well-coordinated team

(Moeller, in press). The roles and responsibilities of each team member should be well defined and clearly understood. Essential team members are families, pediatricians or primary care physicians, audiologists, otolaryngologists, speech-language pathologists, educators of children who are hard of hearing or deaf, and other early intervention professionals involved in delivering EHDI services (Joint Committee of ASHA and Council on Education of the Deaf, 1994). Provisions for supportive family education, counseling, and guidance should be available (Calderon, Bargones, & Sidman, 1998).

Pediatricians and other primary care physicians, working in partnership with parents and other health-care professionals, make up the infant's "medical home." A medical home is defined as an approach to providing health care services where care is accessible, family-centered, continuous, comprehensive, coordinated, compassionate, and culturally competent. Pediatricians act in partnership with parents in a medical home to identify and access services needed in developing a global plan of appropriate and necessary health and habilitative care for infants identified with hearing loss. The infant's pediatrician or other primary care physician functions as the advocate for the whole child within the context of the medical home (American Academy of Pediatrics, 1992, 1993).

As experts in identification, evaluation, and auditory habilitation of infants who are hard of hearing and deaf, audiologists are involved in each component of the EHDI process. For the hearing screening component, audiologists provide program development, management, quality assessment, service coordination, and effective transition to evaluation, habilitative, and intervention services. For the follow-up component, audiologists provide comprehensive audiologic assessment to confirm the existence of the hearing loss, evaluate the infant for candidacy for amplification and other sensory devices and assistive technology, and ensure prompt referral to early intervention programs. For the early intervention component, audiologists provide timely fitting and monitoring of amplification (sensory devices and assistive technology) with family consent, family education, counseling, and ongoing participation in the infant's service plan (Pediatric Working Group of the Conference on Amplification for Children with Auditory Deficits, 1996). In addition, audiologists provide direct auditory habilitation services to infants and families. Audiologists participate in the assessment of candidacy for cochlear implantation.

Otolaryngologists are physicians whose specialty includes the identification, evaluation, and treatment of ear diseases and syndromes related to hearing loss. Families consult an otolaryngologist to determine the etiology of the hearing loss, the presence of related syndromes involving the head and neck structures, and related risk indicators (Section III. E below) for hearing loss. An otolaryngologist with expertise in childhood hearing loss can determine whether medical and/or surgical intervention may be appropriate. When medical and/or surgical intervention is provided, the otolaryngologist is involved in the long-term monitoring and follow-up within the infant's medical home. The otolaryngologist also provides information and participates in the assessment for candidacy for amplification, assistive devices, and cochlear implantation.

Early intervention professionals provide comprehensive family-centered services. They are professionals trained in a variety of academic disciplines, such as speech-language pathology, audiology, education of children who are hard of hearing and deaf, service coordination, or early childhood special education. All individuals who provide services to infants with hearing loss should have training and expertise in auditory, speech, and language development; communication approaches for infants with hearing loss and their families (e.g., cued speech, sign language systems including American Sign Language); and child development (Ross, 1990; Stredler-Brown, 1999). Speech-language pathologists provide both evaluation and treatment for language, speech, and cognitive-communication development (ASHA, 1989). Educators of children who are hard of hearing and deaf integrate the development of communicative competence within the infant's entire development, including a variety of social, linguistic, and cognitive/academic contexts (Joint Committee of ASHA & CED, 1994). In collaboration with the family and other EHDI team members, the service coordinator (case manager) facilitates the family's transition from screening to evaluation to early intervention; links the family to the local Part C system (Public Law 105–17: the amendments to the Individuals with Disabilities Education Act, IDEA, 1997; U.S. Department of Education, Office of Special Education and Rehabilitative Services, 1998); monitors the timeliness of the services; and provides information regarding program options, funding sources, communication choices, and emotional support. This professional incorporates the family's preferences for outcomes into an individualized family service plan (IFSP) as required by federal legislation (IDEA, as defined above). The service coordinator supports the family in stimulation of the infant's communicative development; monitors the infant's progress in language, motor, cognitive and social-emotional development in the IFSP review; and assists the family in advocating for its infant's unique developmental needs.

B. Hearing Screening (Principles 1 and 8)

1. Personnel. Teams of professionals, including audiologists, physicians (neonatologists, pediatricians, other primary care physicians, and otolaryngologists), and nursing personnel, should be involved in establishing the UNHS component of EHDI programs. Hospitals and agencies should designate a physician to oversee the medical aspects of the EHDI program. Audiologists should be designated as the program manager with supervisory responsibilities for the hearing screening and audiologic aspects of the EHDI program and should be involved in the design, implementation, and evaluation of screening programs (including those of small and rural hospitals) (Joint Committee on Infant Hearing, 1994a,b). In addition to audiologists, personnel who carry out the screening procedure may include nurses, speech-language pathologists, and others who are trained by the audiologist (American Academy of Audiology, 1998; American Speech-Language-Hearing Association, 1997; National Institute on Deafness and Other Communication Disorders, 1993, 1997; White & Maxon, 1999).

2. Program Protocol Development. Each team of professionals responsible for the hospital-based UNHS program needs to undertake a comprehensive review of the current hospital infrastructure before implementation of screening. The development of a hospital-based screening program should consider technology, screening protocols including the timing of the screening relative to nursery discharge, availability of qualified screening personnel, acoustically appropriate environments, follow-up referral criteria, information management, and quality control. Reporting and communication management must all be defined. These include the content of reports to physicians and parents, documentation of results in medical records, and methods for reporting to state registries and national data sets. Methods for ensuring that communications to parents are confidential and sensitive should be well defined. Health communication specialists should work with EHDI stakeholders to develop and disseminate family information materials that are accessible and represent the range of alternatives. Materials should be produced in languages other than English for diverse cultures and for low-literacy consumers. Quality indicators and outcome measurements for each component of the UNHS program should be identified and defined before implementation of screening to monitor compliance with program benchmarks. Solutions to problems are often found at the local level. Community resources should be accessed to achieve successful implementation of UNHS.

3. Screening Technologies. Objective physiologic measures must be employed to detect newborns and very young infants with the targeted hearing loss. Current physiologic measures used for detecting unilateral or bilateral hearing loss of various severities include otoacoustic emissions (OAEs), either transient-evoked (TEOAE) or distortion-product (DPOAE), and/or auditory brainstem response (ABR). Both OAE and ABR technologies have been successfully implemented for universal newborn hearing screening (Finitzo, Albright, & O'Neal, 1998; Mason & Hermann, 1998; Vohr, Carty, Moore, & Letourneau, 1998). Both technologies are noninvasive recordings of physiologic activity that underlie normal auditory function and that are easily recorded in neonates. Both OAE and ABR measures are highly correlated with the degree of peripheral hearing sensitivity.

OAEs are sensitive to outer hair cell dysfunction. The technology can be used to detect sensory (i.e., inner ear) hearing loss (Gorga et al., 1993; Prieve et al., 1993). OAEs can be reliably recorded in neonates in response to stimuli in the frequency range above 1500 Hz. The OAE is known to be sensitive to outer ear canal obstruction and middle ear effusion, and, therefore, temporary conductive dysfunction can cause a positive test result (a "refer" outcome) in the presence of normal cochlear function (Doyle, Burggraaff, Fujikawa, Kim, & MacArthur, 1997). Because OAE responses are generated within the cochlea by the outer hair cells, OAE evaluation does not detect neural (i.e., eighth nerve or auditory brainstem pathway) dysfunction. Infants with auditory neuropathy or neural conduction disorders without concomitant sensory (i.e., outer hair cell) dysfunction will not be detected by OAEs.

The ABR reflects activity of the cochlea, auditory nerve, and auditory brainstem pathways. When used as a threshold measure, the click-evoked ABR is highly correlated with hearing sensitivity in the frequency range from 1000 to 8000 Hz (Gorga et al., 1993; Hyde, Riko, & Malizia, 1990). The ABR is sensitive to auditory nerve and brainstem dysfunction; therefore, ABR screening may result in a positive test (a "refer" outcome) in the absence of peripheral (e.g., middle ear or cochlear) hearing loss. Because the ABR is generated by auditory neural pathways, the ABR will detect auditory neuropathy or neural conduction disorders in newborns.

Development of a program includes the establishment of the interpretive criteria for pass and refer. Interpretive criteria should be founded on a clear scientific rationale. Such rationale may be based in statistics and signal detection theory or heuristic and empirically derived. Test performance efficiency, including sensitivity, specificity, and the positive and negative predictive values, should be evidenced-based (Hyde, Davidson, & Alberti, 1991; Hyde, Sininger, & Don, 1998). Screening technologies that incorporate automated response detection are preferred over those that require operator interpretation and decision making. Automated algorithms eliminate the need for individual test interpretation, reduce the effects of screener bias and errors on test outcome, and ensure test consistency across all infants, test conditions, and screening personnel (Eilers, Miskiel, Ozdamar, Urbano, & Widen, 1991; Herrmann, Thornton, & Joseph, 1995; McFarland, Simmons, & Jones, 1980; Ozdamar, Delgado, Eilers, & Urbano, 1994; Pool & Finitzo, 1989). Programs that use trained and supervised nonprofessional staff must use technologies that provide automated pass-refer criteria. Before incorporating automated response detection algorithms, however, the screening program must ensure that the algorithms have been validated by rigorous scientific methods and that those results have been reported in peer-reviewed publications.

Some infants with hearing loss will pass the newborn hearing screening. Both ABR and OAE technology can show false-negative findings, depending on whether hearing loss exists in configurations that include normal hearing for one or more frequencies in the target range. These would include isolated low-frequency (i.e., below 1000 Hz) hearing loss or steeply sloping high-frequency (i.e., above 2000 Hz) hearing loss. ABR can show false-negative findings with midfrequency hearing loss (i.e., 500–2000 Hz). Additional variables that influence screening test performance include the population (age and presence of risk indicators), the targeted hearing loss, the performance and recording characteristics of the test technology, the pass-refer criteria, and excessive retesting using the same technology (which increases the likelihood of a false-negative screening outcome).

4. Screening Protocols. A variety of hospital-based UNHS screening protocols have been successfully implemented that permit all newborns access to hearing screening during their birth admission (Arehart, Yoshinaga-Itano, Thomson, V., Gabbard, & Stredler Brown, 1998; Finitzo, Albright, & O'Neal, 1998; Gravel et al., 2000; Mason & Hermann, 1998; Mehl & Thomson, 1998; Vohr, Carty, Moore, & Letourneau, 1998). Most infants pass their initial screening test. Many inpatient-screening protocols provide one or more repeat screens, using the same or a different technology, if the newborn does not pass the initial birth screen. For example, hospitals may screen with OAE technology or ABR technology and retest infants who "refer" with the same or the other technology.

Some screening protocols incorporate an outpatient rescreening of infants who do not pass the birth admission screening within 1 month of hospital discharge. The mechanism of rescreening an infant minimizes the number of false-positive referrals for follow-up audiologic and medical evaluation. Outpatient screening by 1 month of age should also be available to infants who were discharged before receiving the birth admission screening or who were born outside a hospital or birthing center.

5. *Benchmarks and Quality Indicators for Birth Admission Hearing Screening.*

(a) Recommended UNHS benchmarks include the following:

(1) Within 6 months of program initiation, hospitals or birthing centers screen a minimum of 95% of infants during their birth admission or before 1 month of age. Programs can achieve and maintain this outcome despite birth admissions of 24 or fewer hours (Finitzo, Albright, & O'Neal, 1998; Mason & Hermann, 1998; Spivak et al., 2000; Vohr, Carty, Moore, & Letourneau, 1998).

(2) The referral rate for audiologic and medical evaluation following the screening process (in-hospital during birth admission or during both birth admission and outpatient follow-up screening) should be 4% or less within 1 year of program initiation.

(3) The agency within the EHDI program with defined responsibility for follow-up (often a state department of health) documents efforts to obtain follow-up on a minimum of 95% of infants who do not pass the hearing screening. Ideally, a program should achieve a return-for-follow-up of 70% of infants or more (Prieve et al., 2000). Successful follow-up is influenced by such factors as lack of adequate tracking information, changes in the names or addresses of mother and/or infant, absence of a designated medical home for the infant, and lack of health insurance that covers follow-up services.

(b) Associated quality indicators of the screening component of EHDI programs may include the following:

(1) Percentage of infants screened during the birth admission.

(2) Percentage of infants screened before 1 month of age.

(3) Percentage of infants who do not pass the birth admission screen.

(4) Percentage of infants who do not pass the birth admission screening who return for follow-up services (either outpatient screening and/or audiologic and medical evaluation).

(5) Percentage of infants who do not pass the birth admission/outpatient screen(s) who are referred for audiologic and medical evaluation.

(6) Percentage of families who refuse hearing screening on birth admission.

Quality indicators for hospital-based programs should be monitored monthly to ascertain whether a program is achieving expected benchmarks and outcomes (targets and goals). Frequent measures of quality permit prompt recognition and correction of any unstable component of the screening process (Agency for Healthcare Policy and Research, 1995). Focused reeducation for staff can be undertaken in a timely manner to address strategies to achieve targets and goals.

C. Confirmation of Hearing Loss in Infants Referred From UNHS (Principles 2 and 8)

Infants who meet the defined criteria for referral should receive follow-up audiologic and medical evaluations before 3 months of age. The infant should be referred for comprehensive audiologic assessment and specialty medical evaluations to confirm the presence of hearing loss and to determine type, nature, options for treatment, and (whenever possible) etiology of the hearing loss. After a hearing loss is confirmed, coordination of services should be expedited by the infant's medical home and Individuals with Disabilities Education Act (IDEA) Part C coordinating agencies. Part C agencies are responsible for Child Find and intervention for children with disabilities and the related professionals with expertise in hearing loss evaluation and treatment. The infant's primary care physician, with guidance or coordination from state and local agencies, should address parental concerns and mobilize systems on behalf of the infant and family. Professionals in health care and education must interface to provide families with needed services for the infant with hearing loss.

1. Audiologic Evaluation. Audiologists providing the initial audiologic test battery to confirm the existence of a hearing loss in infants must include physiologic measures and developmentally appropriate behavioral techniques. Adequate confirmation of an infant's hearing status cannot be obtained from a single test measure. Rather, a test battery is required to cross-check results of both behavioral and physiologic measures (Jerger & Hayes, 1976). The purpose of the audiologic test battery is to assess the integrity of the auditory system, to estimate hearing sensitivity, and to identify all intervention options. Regardless of the infant's age, ear-specific estimates of type, degree, and configuration of hearing loss should be obtained.

For infants birth to 6 months of age, the test battery should begin with a child and family history and must include an electrophysiologic measure of threshold such as ABR (Sininger, Abdala, & Cone-Wesson, 1997; Stapells, Gravel, & Martin, 1995) or other appropriate electrophysiologic tests (Rance, Rickards, Cohen, DeVidi, & Clark, 1995) using frequency-specific stimuli. The assessment of the young infant must include OAEs (Prieve, Fitzgerald, Schulte, & Demp, 1997), a measure of middle ear function, acoustic reflex thresholds, observation of the infant's behavioral response to sound, and parental report of emerging communication and auditory behaviors. Appropriate measures of middle ear function for this age group include reflectance (Keefe & Levi, 1996), tympanometry using appropriate frequency probe stimuli (Marchant et al., 1986), bone conduction ABR (Cone-Wesson & Ramirez, 1997), and/or pneumatic otoscopy.

The confirmatory audiologic test battery for infants and toddlers age 6 through 36 months includes a child and family history, behavioral response audiometry (either visual reinforcement or conditioned play audiometry depending on the child's developmental age), OAEs, acoustic immittance measures (including acoustic reflex thresholds), speech detection and recognition measures (Diefendorf & Gravel, 1996; Gravel & Hood, 1999), parental report of auditory and visual behaviors, and a screening of the infant's communication milestones. Physiologic tests, such as ABR, should be performed at least during the initial evaluation to confirm type, degree, and configuration of hearing loss.

In accordance with IDEA, referral to a public agency must take place within 2 working days after the infant has been identified as needing evaluation. Once the public agency receives the referral, its role is to appoint a service coordinator, identify an audiologist to complete the audiologic evaluation, and identify other qualified personnel to determine the child's level of functioning. An IFSP must be held within 45 days of receiving the referral (Public Law 105–17: the amendments to the Individuals with Disabilities Education Act, IDEA 1997; U.S. Department of Education, Office of Special Education and Rehabilitative Services, 1998).

2. Medical Evaluation. Every infant with confirmed hearing loss and/or middle ear dysfunction should be referred for otologic and other medical evaluation. The purpose of these evaluations is to determine the etiology of hearing loss, to identify related physical conditions, and to provide recommendations for medical treatment as well as referral for other services. Essential components of the medical evaluation include clinical history, family history, and physical examination as well as indicated laboratory and radiologic studies. When indicated and with family consent, the otolaryngologist may consult with a geneticist for chromosome analysis and for evaluation of specific syndromes related to hearing loss.

(a) Pediatrician or primary care physician: The infant's pediatrician or other primary care physician is responsible for monitoring the general health and well-being of the infant. In addition, the primary care physician in partnership with the family and other health care professionals, assures that audiologic assessment is conducted on infants who do not pass screening and initiates referrals for medical specialty evaluations necessary to determine the etiology of the hearing loss. Middle-ear status should be monitored because the presence of middle-ear effusion can further compromise hearing. The pediatrician or primary care physician should review the infant's history for presence of risk indicators that require monitoring for delayed onset and/or progressive hearing loss and should insure periodic audiologic evaluation for children at risk. Also, because 30% to 40% of children with confirmed hearing loss will demonstrate developmental delays or other disabilities, the primary care physician should monitor developmental milestones and initiate referrals related to suspected disabilities (Karchmer & Allen, 1999).

(b) Otolaryngologist: The otolaryngologist's evaluation should consist of a comprehensive clinical history; family history; physical assessment, and laboratory tests involving the ears, head, face, neck, and such other systems as skin (pigmentation), eye, heart, kidney, and thyroid that could be affected by childhood hearing loss (Tomaski & Grundfast, 1999). The physical examination of the ear involves identification of external ear malformations including preauricular tags and sinuses, abnormalities or obstruction of ear canals such as the presence of excessive cerumen, and abnormalities of the tympanic membrane and/or middle ear, including otitis media with effusion. Supplementary evaluations may include imaging studies of the temporal bones and electrocardiograms. Laboratory assessments useful for identifying etiology may include urinalysis, blood tests for congenital or early-onset infection (e.g., cytomegalovirus, syphilis, toxoplasmosis), and specimen analyses for genetic conditions associated with hearing loss.

(c) Other medical specialists: The etiology of neonatal hearing loss may remain uncertain in as many as 30% to 40% of children. However, most congenital hearing loss is hereditary, and nearly 200 syndromic and nonsyndromic forms have already been identified (Brookhouser, Worthington, & Kelly, 1994). For 20% to 30% of children, there are associated clinical findings that can be of importance in patient management. Where thorough physical and laboratory investigations fail to define the etiology of hearing loss, families should be offered the option of genetic evaluation and counseling by a medical geneticist. The medical geneticist is responsible for the collection and interpretation of family history data, the clinical evaluation and diagnosis of inherited diseases, the performance and assessment of genetic tests, and the provision of genetic counseling. Geneticists are qualified to interpret the significance and limitations of new tests and to convey the current status of knowledge during genetic counseling.

Other medical specialty areas, including developmental pediatrics, neurology, ophthalmology, cardiology and nephrology, may be consulted to determine the presence of related body-system disorders as part of syndromes associated with hearing loss. In addition, every infant with hearing loss should receive an ophthalmologic evaluation at regular intervals to rule out concomitant late-onset vision disorders (Gallaudet University Center for Assessment and Demographic Study, 1998; Johnson, 1999). Many infants with hearing loss will have received care in an NICU. Because NICU-enrolled infants will demonstrate other developmental disorders, the assistance of a developmental pediatrician may be valuable for management of these infants.

3. Benchmarks and quality indicators for the confirmation of hearing loss.
(a) Benchmarks
There are few published data available to provide targets for programs involved in confirmation of hearing loss. Until benchmark data that provide a goal are published, programs should strive to provide care to 100% of infants needing services.

1. Comprehensive services for infants and families referred following screening are coordinated between the infant's medical home, family, and related professionals with expertise in hearing loss and the state and local agencies responsible for provision of services to children with hearing loss.

2. Infants referred from UNHS begin audiologic and medical evaluations before 3 months of age or 3 months after discharge for NICU infants (Dalzell et al., 2000).

3. Infants with evidence of hearing loss on audiologic assessment receive an otologic evaluation.

4. Families and professionals perceive the medical and audiologic evaluation process as positive and supportive.

5. Families receive referral to Part C coordinating agencies, appropriate intervention programs, parent/consumer and professional organizations, and child-find coordinators if necessary.

(b) Associated quality indicators of the confirmation of hearing loss component of the EHDI programs may include the following:

1. Percentage of infants and families whose care is coordinated between the medical home and related professionals.

2. Percentage of infants whose audiologic and medical evaluations are obtained before an infant is 3 months of age.

3. Percentage of infants with confirmed hearing loss referred for otologic evaluation.

4. Percentage of families who accept audiologic and medical evaluation services.

5. Percentage of families of infants with confirmed hearing loss that have a signed IFSP by the time the infant reaches 6 months of age.

D. Early Intervention (Principles 3 and 8)

The mounting evidence for the crucial nature of early experience in brain development provides the impetus to ensure learning opportunities for all infants (Kuhl et al., 1997; Kuhl, Williams, Lacerda, Stevens, & Lindblom, 1992; Sininger, Doyle, & Moore, 1999). Research demonstrates that intensive early intervention can alter positively the cognitive and developmental outcomes of young infants with disabilities or infants who are socially and economically disadvantaged (Guralnick, 1997; Infant Health and Development Program, 1990; Ramey & Ramey, 1992, 1998). Yoshinaga-Itano, Sedey, Coulter, and Mehl (1998), Moeller (in press), and Carney and Moeller (1998) have corroborated these findings in infants with hearing loss.

1. Early Intervention Program Development. Early intervention services should be designed to meet the individualized needs of the infant and family, including addressing acquisition of communicative competence, social skills, emotional well-being, and positive self-esteem (Karchmer & Allen, 1999). Six frequently cited principles of effective early intervention are (1) developmental timing, (2) program intensity, (3) direct learning, (4) program breadth and flexibility, (5) recognition of individual differences, and (6) environmental support and family involvement (Meadow-Orleans, Mertens, Sass-Lehrer, & Scott-Olson, 1997; Moeller & Condon, 1994; Ramey & Ramey, 1992, 1998; Stredler-Brown, 1998; Thomblin, Spencer, Flock, Tyler, & Gantz, 1999).

Developmental timing refers to the age at which services begin and the duration of enrollment. Programs that enroll infants at younger ages and continue longer are found to produce the greatest benefits. Program intensity refers to the amount of intervention and is measured by multiple factors, such as the number of home visits/contacts per week for the infant and the family's participation in intervention. Greater developmental progress occurs when the infant and family are actively and regularly involved in the intervention. The principle of direct learning encompasses the idea that center-based and home-based learning experiences are more effective when there is direct (provided by trained professionals) as well as indirect intervention. The principle of program breadth and flexibility notes that successful intervention programs offer a broad spectrum of services and are flexible and multifaceted to meet the unique needs of the infant and family. Rates of progress and benefits from programs are functions of infant and family individual differences; not everyone progresses at the same rate nor benefits from programs to the same extent. Finally, the benefits of early intervention continue over time depending on the effectiveness of existing supports: family involvement and other environmental supports (e.g., home, school, health, and peer) (Ramey & Ramey, 1992). Individualization in intervention tailors the services to be developmentally appropriate and recognizes meaningful individual and family differences (Cohen, 1993, 1997).

Optimal intervention strategies for the infant with any hearing loss require that intervention begin as soon as there is confirmation of a permanent hearing loss to enhance the child's acquisition of developmentally appropriate language skills. All infants with the targeted hearing loss are at risk for delayed communication development and should receive early intervention services (Bess, Dodd-Murphy, & Parker, 1998; Rushmer, 1992). Early intervention provides appropriate services for the child with hearing loss and assures that families receive consumer-oriented information. Documented discussion must occur about the full range of resources in early intervention and education programs for children with hearing loss.

In supplying information to families, professionals must recognize and respect the family's natural transitions through the grieving process at the time of initial diagnosis of hearing loss and at different intervention decision-making stages (Cherow, Dickman, & Epstein, 1999; Luterman, 1985; Luterman & Kurtzer-White, 1999). The range of intervention options should be reviewed at least every 6 months. Families should be apprised of individuals who and organizations that can enhance informed decision-making such as peer models, persons who are hard of hearing and deaf, and consumer and professional associations (Baker-Hawkins & Easterbrooks, 1994; Cherow, Dickman, & Epstein, 1999).

Early intervention must be preceded by a comprehensive assessment of the infant's and family's needs and the family's informed decision-making related to those needs (Stredler-Brown & Yoshinaga-Itano, 1994). Federal law provides funds for states to participate in early intervention services for infants with hearing loss (Public Law 105–17: the amendments to the Individuals with Disabilities Education Act, IDEA 1997; U.S. Department of Education, Office of Special Education and Rehabilitative Services, 1998). Part C of IDEA requires that an interdisciplinary developmental evaluation be completed to determine the child's level of functioning in each of the following developmental areas: cognitive, physical, and communicative development; social or emotional development; and adaptive development (34 C.F.R. Part 303 ß303.322). The IFSP is to be developed by the family and service coordinator (Joint Committee of ASHA and Council on Education of the Deaf, 1994). The IFSP specifies needs, outcomes, intervention components, and anticipated developmental progress. The full evaluation process must be completed within 45 days of primary referral. However, intervention services may commence before completion of the full evaluation of all developmental areas and during the confirmation of the hearing loss if parent/guardian consent is obtained and an interim IFSP is developed (Matkin, 1988). Once services are begun, ongoing assessment of progress is crucial to determine appropriateness of the intervention strategies. In addition, the family and service coordinator must review the IFSP at least every 6 months to determine whether progress toward achieving the outcomes is being made and whether the outcomes should be modified or revised. The IFSP must be evaluated at least annually and—taking into consideration the results of any current evaluations, progress made, and other new information, revised as appropriate (34 CFR Part 303 ß303.342).

Thirty to 40% of children with hearing loss demonstrate additional disabilities that may have concomitant effects on communication and related development (Gallaudet University Center for Assessment and Demographic Study, 1998; Schildroth & Hotto, 1993). Thus, interdisciplinary assessment and intervention are essential to address the developmental needs of all children who are hard of hearing or deaf, especially those with additional developmental disabilities (Cherow, Dickman, & Epstein, 1999; Cherow, Matkin, & Trybus, 1985).

The diverse demographics of infants with hearing loss and their families highlight the importance of shaping the early intervention curriculum to the infant and family profile (Calderon, Bargones, & Sidman, 1998; Karchmer & Allen, 1999). Families who live in underserved areas may have less accessibility, fewer professional resources, deaf or hard of hearing role models, or sign language interpreters available to assist them. A growing number of children with hearing loss in the United States are from families that are non-native English speaking (Baker-Hawkins & Easterbrooks, 1994; Christensen & Delgado, 1993;

Cohen, 1997; Cohen, Fischgrund, & Redding, 1990; Scott, 1998). These factors underscore the necessity of providing comprehensive, culturally sensitive information to families—information that is responsive to their needs and that results in informed choices (Schwartz, 1996).

2. *Audiologic Habilitation.* The vast majority of infants and children with bilateral hearing loss benefit from some form of personal amplification or sensory device (Pediatric Working Group of the Conference on Amplification for Children with Auditory Deficits, 1996). If the family chooses individualized personal amplification for their infant, hearing aid selection and fitting should be provided by the audiologist in a timely fashion. Delay between confirmation of the hearing loss and amplification should be minimized (Arehart, Yoshinaga-Itano, Thomson, Gabbard, & Stredler Brown, 1998).

Hearing aid fitting proceeds optimally when the results of the medical evaluation and physiologic (OAE and ABR) and behavioral audiologic assessments are in accord. However, the provision of amplification should proceed based on physiologic measures alone if behavioral measures of threshold are precluded because of the infant's age or developmental level. In such cases, behavioral measures should be obtained as soon as possible to corroborate the physiologic findings. The goal of amplification fitting is to provide the infant with maximum access to the acoustic features of speech within a listening range that is safe and comfortable. That is, amplified speech should be comfortably above the infant's sensory threshold, but below the level of discomfort across the speech frequency range for both ears (Pediatric Working Group of the Conference on Amplification for Children with Auditory Deficits, 1996).

The amplification fitting protocol should combine prescriptive procedures that incorporate individual real-ear measurements (Pediatric Working Group of the Conference on Amplification for Children with Auditory Deficits, 1996). These techniques allow amplification to be individually fitted to meet the unique characteristics of each infant's hearing loss. Validation of the benefits of amplification, particularly for speech perception, should be examined in the infant's typical listening environments. Complementary or alternative sensory technology (FM systems, vibrotactile aids, or cochlear implants) may be recommended as the primary and/or secondary listening device, depending on the degree of the infant's hearing loss, goals of auditory habilitation, acoustic environments, and family's informed choices (ASHA, 1991). Long-term monitoring of personal amplification requires audiologic assessment; electroacoustic, real-ear, and functional checks of the amplification/listening device, as well as refinement of the prescriptive targets. Long-term monitoring also includes continual validation of communication, social-emotional, cognitive, and later academic development to assure that progress is commensurate with the infant's abilities. The latter data are obtained through interdisciplinary evaluation and collaboration by the IFSP team that includes the family.

The impact of otitis media with effusion (OME) is greater for infants with sensorineural hearing loss than those with normal cochlear function. Sensory or permanent conductive hearing loss is compounded by additional conductive hearing loss associated with OME. OME further reduces access to auditory/oral language stimulation and spoken language development for infants whose families choose an auditory-oral approach to communication development. Prompt referral to otolaryngologists for treatment of persistent or recurrent OME is indicated in infants with sensorineural hearing loss. Ongoing medical/surgical management of OME may be needed to resolve the condition. Management of OME, however, should not delay the prompt fitting of amplification unless there are medical contraindications (Brookhouser, Worthington, & Kelly, 1994).

3. *Medical and Surgical Intervention.* Medical intervention is the process by which a physician provides medical diagnosis and direction for medical and/or surgical treatment options for hearing loss and/or related medical disorder(s) associated with hearing loss. Treatment varies from the removal of cerumen and the treatment of otitis media with effusion to long-term plans for reconstructive surgery and assessment of candidacy for cochlear implants. If necessary, surgical treatment of malformation of the outer and middle ears should be considered in the intervention plan for infants with conductive or sensorineural plus conductive hearing loss. Cochlear implants may be an option for certain children age 12 months and older with profound hearing loss who show limited benefit from conventional amplifications. As noted above, in infants with identified sensorineural hearing loss, the presence of otitis media needs to be recognized promptly and treated, with the infant monitored on a periodic basis.

4. *Communication Assessment and Intervention.* Language is acquired with greater ease during certain sensitive periods of infants' and toddlers' development (Clark, 1994; Mahshie, 1995). The process of language acquisition includes learning the precursors of language, such as the rules pertaining to selective attention and turn taking (Kuhl et al., 1997; Kuhl, Williams, Lacerda, Stevens, & Lindblom, 1992). Cognitive, social, and emotional developments depend on the acquisition of language. Development in these areas is synergistic. A complete language evaluation should be performed for infants and toddlers with hearing loss. The evaluation should include an assessment of oral, manual, and/or visual mechanisms as well as cognitive abilities.

A primary focus of early intervention programs is to support families in developing the communication abilities of their infants and toddlers who are hard of hearing or deaf (Carney & Moeller, 1998). Elements of oral and sign language development include vocal/manual babbling, vocal/visual turn-taking, and early word/sign acquisition. Oral and/or sign language development should be commensurate with the child's age and cognitive abilities and should include acquisition of phonologic (for spoken language), visual/spatial/motor (for signed language), morphologic, semantic, syntactic, and pragmatic skills.

Early interventionists should follow family-centered principles to assist in developing communicative competence of infants and toddlers who are hard of hearing or deaf (Baker-Hawkins and Easterbrooks, 1994; Bamford, 1998; Fisher, 1994). Families should be provided with information specific to language development and with family-involved activities that facilitate language development. Early interventionists should ensure access to peer and language models. Peer models might include families with normal hearing children as well as children or adults who are hard of hearing and deaf as appropriate to the needs of the infant with hearing loss (Marschark, 1997; Thompson, 1994). Depending on informed family choices, peer models could include users of visual language (e.g., American Sign Language) and other signed systems as well as users of auditory/oral communication methods for spoken language development

(Pollack, Goldberg, & Coleffe-Schenck, 1997). Information on visual communication methods such as American Sign Language, other signed systems, and cued speech should be provided. Information on oral/auditory language, personal hearing aids, and assistive devices such as FM systems, tactile aids, and cochlear implants should also be made available.

The specific goals of early intervention are to facilitate developmentally appropriate language skills, enhance the family's understanding of its infant's strengths and needs, and promote the family's ability to advocate for its infant. Early intervention should also build family support and confidence in parenting the infant who is deaf or hard of hearing and increase the family's satisfaction with the EHDI process (Fisher, 1994; U.S. Department of Education, Office of Special Education and Rehabilitative Services, 1998). Provision of early intervention services includes monitoring participation and progress of the infant and family as well as adapting and modifying interventions as needed. Systematic documentation of the intervention approach facilitates decision-making on program changes.

5. *Benchmarks and Quality Indicators for Early Intervention Programs.*

(a) Benchmarks

It should be the goal of the intervention component of an EHDI program that all infants be served as described below. Because specific benchmarks for early intervention have yet to be reported, target percentages are not noted here. The JCIH strongly recommends that these data be obtained so that benchmarks may be made available.

1. Infants with hearing loss are enrolled in a family-centered early intervention program before 6 months of age.

2. Infants with hearing loss are enrolled in a family-centered early intervention program with professional personnel who are knowledgeable about the communication needs of infants with hearing loss.

3. Infants with hearing loss and no medical contraindication begin use of amplification when appropriate and agreed on by the family within 1 month of confirmation of the hearing loss.

4. Infants with amplification receive ongoing audiologic monitoring at intervals not to exceed 3 months.

5. Infants enrolled in early intervention achieve language development in the family's chosen communication mode that is commensurate with the infant's developmental level as documented in the IFSP and that is similar to that for hearing peers of a comparable developmental age.

6. Families participate in and express satisfaction with self-advocacy.

(b) Quality indicators for the intervention services may include the following:

1. Percentage of infants with hearing loss who are enrolled in a family-centered early intervention program before 6 months of age

2. Percentage of infants with hearing loss who are enrolled in an early intervention program with professional personnel who are knowledgeable about overall child development as well as the communication needs and intervention options for infants with hearing loss

3. Percentage of infants in early intervention who receive language evaluations at 6-month intervals

4. Percentage of infants and toddlers whose language levels, whether spoken or signed, are commensurate with those of their hearing peers

5. Percentage of infants and families who achieve the outcomes identified on their IFSP

6. Percentage of infants with hearing loss and no medical contraindication who begin use of amplification when agreed on by the family within 1 month of confirmation of the hearing loss

7. Percentage of infants with amplification who receive ongoing audiologic monitoring at intervals not to exceed 3 months.

8. Number of follow-up visits for amplification monitoring and adjustment within the first year following amplification fitting

9. Percentage of families who refuse early intervention services

10. Percentage of families who participate in and express satisfaction with self-advocacy

E. Continued Surveillance of Infants and Toddlers (Principle 4)

Since 1972, the JCIH has identified specific risk indicators that often are associated with infant and childhood hearing loss. These risk indicators have been applied both in the United States and in other countries and serve two purposes. First, risk indicators help identify infants who should receive audiologic evaluation and who live in geographic locations (e.g., developing nations, remote areas) where universal hearing screening is not yet available. The JCIH no longer recommends programs calling for screening at-risk infants because such programs will identify approximately 50% of infants with hearing loss; however, these programs may be useful where resources limit the development of universal newborn hearing screening. Second, because normal hearing at birth does not preclude delayed onset or acquired hearing loss, risk indicators help identify infants who should receive on-going audiologic and medical monitoring and surveillance.

Risk indicators can be divided into two categories: those present during the neonatal period and those that may develop as a result of certain medical conditions or essential medical interventions in the treatment of an ill child. Risk indicators published in the 1994 Position Statement are revised in 2000 to take account of current information. Specifically, data have been considered from an epidemiological study of permanent childhood hearing impairment in the Trent Region of Great Britain from 1985 through 1993 (Fortnum & Davis, 1997) and the recent NIH multicenter study, "Identification of Neonatal Hearing Impairment" (Norton et al., in press). Cone-Wesson et al. (in press) analyzed the prevalence of risk indicators for infants identified with hearing loss in that study. Three thousand one hundred thirty-four infants evaluated during their initial birth hospitalization were reevaluated for the presence of hearing loss between 8 and 12 months of age. The majority of these infants were NICU graduates (2,847), and the remaining 287 infants had risk indicators for hearing loss that did not require intensive care, such as family history or craniofacial anomalies. Infants with history or evidence of transient middle ear dysfunction were excluded from the final analysis, revealing 56 with permanent hearing loss.

Cone-Wesson et al. (in press) determined the prevalence of hearing loss for each risk factor by dividing the number of infants with the risk factor and hearing loss by the total number of infants in the sample with a given risk factor. Hearing loss was present in 11.7% of infants with syndromes associated with hearing loss, which included Trisomy 21; Pierre Robin syndrome; CHARGE syndrome; choanal atresia; Rubinstein-Taybi syndrome; Stickler syndrome; and oculo-auriculo-vertebral (OAV) spectrum (also known as Goldenhar syndrome). Family history of hearing loss had a prevalence of 6.6%, meningitis 5.5%, and craniofacial anomalies 4.7%. In contrast, infants treated with aminogycoside antibiotics had a prevalence of hearing loss of only 1.5%, consistent with data of Finitzo-Hieber, McCracken, & Brown (1985). Analyzing risk indicators, such as ototoxicity, by prevalence points out that although a large number of NICU infants with hearing loss have a history of aminogycoside treatment, only a small percentage of those receiving potentially ototoxic antibiotics actually incurred hearing loss. In fact, 45% of infants treated in the NICU received such treatment (Vohr et al., in press).

1. Given these current data, the JCIH risk indicators have been modified for use in neonates (birth through age 28 days) where universal hearing screening is not yet available. These indicators are as follows:

(a) An illness or condition requiring admission of 48 hours or greater to a NICU (Cone-Wesson et al., in press; Fortnum & Davis, 1997).

(b) Stigmata or other findings associated with a syndrome known to include a sensorineural and or conductive hearing loss (Cone-Wesson et al., in press).

(c) Family history of permanent childhood sensorineural hearing loss (Cone-Wesson et al., in press; Fortnum & Davis, 1997).

(d) Craniofacial anomalies, including those with morphological abnormalities of the pinna and ear canal (Cone-Wesson et al., in press; Fortnum & Davis, 1997).

(e) In utero infection such as cytomegalovirus, herpes, toxoplasmosis, or rubella (Demmler, 1991; Littman, Demmler, Williams, Istas, & Griesser, 1995; Williamson, Demmler, Percy, & Catlin, 1992).

Interpretation of the Cone-Wesson et al. (in press) data reveals that 1 of 56 infants identified with permanent hearing loss revealed clear evidence of late-onset hearing loss by 1 year of age. The definition of late-onset hearing loss for this analysis was a present ABR at 30 dB in the newborn period and hearing thresholds by visual reinforcement audiometry at age 8–12 months 40 dB for all stimuli. The infant with late-onset loss passed screening ABR, TOAE, and DPOAE during the newborn period but had reliable behavioral thresholds revealing a severe hearing loss at 1 year of age. Risk indicators for this infant included low birthweight, respiratory distress syndrome, bronchio-pulmonary dysplasia, and 36 days of mechanical ventilation. Although these data are valuable, additional study of large samples of infants is needed before risk indicators for progressive or delayed-onset hearing loss can be clearly defined.

2. The JCIH recommends the following indicators for use with neonates or infants (29 days through 2 years). These indicators place an infant at risk for progressive or delayed-onset sensorineural hearing loss and/or conductive hearing loss. Any infant with these risk indicators for progressive or delayed-onset hear-

ing loss who has passed the birth screen should, nonetheless, receive audiologic monitoring every 6 months until age 3 years. These indicators are as follows:

(a) Parental or caregiver concern regarding hearing, speech, language, and or developmental delay.

(b) Family history of permanent childhood hearing loss (Grundfast, 1996).

(c) Stigmata or other findings associated with a syndrome known to include a sensorineural or conductive hearing loss or eustachian tube dysfunction.

(d) Postnatal infections associated with sensorineural hearing loss including bacterial meningitis (Ozdamar, Kraus, & Stein, 1983).

(e) In utero infections such as cytomegalovirus, herpes, rubella, syphilis, and toxoplasmosis.

(f) Neonatal indicators—specifically hyperbilirubinemia at a serum level requiring exchange transfusion, persistent pulmonary hypertension of the newborn associated with mechanical ventilation, and conditions requiring the use of extracorporeal membrane oxygenation (ECMO) (Roizen, 1999).

(g) Syndromes associated with progressive hearing loss such as neurofibromatosis, osteopetrosis, and Usher's syndrome.

(h) Neurodegenerative disorders, such as Hunter syndrome, or sensory motor neuropathies, such as Friedreich's ataxia and Charcot-Marie-Tooth syndrome.

(i) Head trauma.

(j) Recurrent or persistent otitis media with effusion for at least 3 months (Stool et al. 1994).

Because some important indicators, such as family history of hearing loss, may not be determined during the course of UNHS programs, the presence of all late-onset risk indicators should be determined in the medical home during early well-baby visits. Those infants with significant late-onset risk factors should be carefully monitored for normal communication developmental milestones during routine medical care.

The JCIH recommends ongoing audiologic and medical monitoring of infants with unilateral, mild, or chronic conductive hearing loss. Infants and children with mild or unilateral hearing loss may also experience adverse speech, language, and communication skill development, as well as difficulties with social, emotional, and educational development (Bess, Dodd-Murphy, & Parker, 1998; Blair, Petterson, & Viehweg, 1985; Davis, Elfenbein, Schum, & Bentler, 1986; Matkin & Bess, 1998; Roush & Matkin, 1994; Tharpe & Bess, 1995). Infants with unilateral hearing loss are at risk for progressive and/or bilateral hearing loss (Brookhouser, Worthington, & Kelly, 1994). Infants with frequent episodes of OME also require additional vigilance to address the potential adverse effects of fluctuating conductive hearing loss associated with persistent or recurrent OME (Friel-Patti & Finitzo, 1990; Friel-Patti, Finitzo, Meyerhoff, & Hieber, 1986; Friel-Patti, Finitzo-Hieber, Conti, & Brown, 1982; Gravel & Wallace, 1992; Jerger, Jerger, Alford, & Abrams, 1983; Roberts, Burchinal, & Medley, 1995; Stool et al., 1994; Wallace et al., 1988).

The population of infants cared for in the NICU may also be at increased risk for neural conduction and/or auditory brainstem dysfunction, including auditory neuropathy. Auditory neuropathy is a recently identified disorder, characterized by a unique constellation of behavioral and physiologic auditory test results (Gravel & Stapells, 1993; Kraus, Ozdamar, Stein, & Reed, 1984; Sininger, Hood, Starr, Berlin, & and Picton, 1995; Starr, Picton, Sininger, Hood, & Berlin, 1996; Stein et al., 1996). Behaviorally, children with auditory neuropathy have been reported to exhibit mild-to-profound hearing loss and poor speech perception. Physiologic measures of auditory function (e.g., otoacoustic emissions and auditory brainstem response) demonstrate the finding of normal OAEs (suggesting normal outer hair cell function) and atypical or absent ABRs (suggesting neural conduction dysfunction). Reports suggest that those at increased risk for auditory neuropathy are (a) infants with a compromised neonatal course who receive intensive neonatal care (Berlin et al., 1999; Stein et al., 1996), (b) children with a family history of childhood hearing loss (Corley & Crabbe, 1999), and (c) infants with hyperbilirubinemia (Stein et al., 1996). Currently, neither the prevalence of auditory neuropathy in newborns nor the natural history of the disorder is known, and treatment options are not well defined. Audiologic and medical monitoring of infants at risk for auditory neuropathy is recommended. Infants with these disorders can be detected only by the use of OAE and ABR technology used in combination. Prospective investigations of this neural conduction disorder are warranted (see Future Directions).

F. Protection of Infants' and Families' Rights (Principles 5 and 6)

Each agency or institution involved in the EHDI process shares the responsibility for protecting infant and family rights. These rights include access to UNHS, information in the family's native language, choice, and confidentiality (NIDCD, 1999). Families should receive information about childhood hearing loss in consumer-oriented language. The information should cover the prevalence and effects of early hearing loss, the potential benefits and risks of screening and evaluation procedures, and the prognosis with and without early identification and intervention. Alternative funding sources should be sought if the parent(s) or legal guardian desires to have the infant screened for hearing loss but does not have a reimbursement option.

Families have the same right to accept or decline hearing screening or any follow-up care for their newborn as they do any other screening or evaluation procedures or intervention. Implied or written consent consistent with the protocol of the hospital or the requirements of the state should be obtained for newborn hearing screening after determining the family or legal guardian have been provided appropriate educational materials and have had their questions answered by qualified health care personnel.

The results of screening are to be communicated verbally and in writing to families by health care professionals knowledgeable about hearing loss and the appropriate interpretation of the screening results. EHDI data merit the same level of confidentiality and security afforded all other health care and education information in practice and law. The newborn and his or her family have the right to confidentiality of the screening and follow-up assessments and the acceptance or rejection of suggested intervention(s). Consent of the parent or guardian is the basic legal requisite for disclosure of medical information. In compliance with federal and state laws, mechanisms should be established that assure parental release and approval of all communications regarding the infant's test results, including those to the infant's medical home and early intervention coordinating agency and programs. Confidentiality requires that family and infant information not be transmitted or accessible in unsecured data formats. An effective information system is a tool to assure both proper communication and confidentiality of EHDI information.

G. Information Infrastructure (Principles 7 and 8)

In concert with the 1994 Position Statement (JCIH, 1994a,b), the JCIH recommends development of uniform state registries and national information databases incorporating standardized methodology, reporting, and system evaluation. The choice of an information management system affects what questions can be answered and what tools are available for infant and family management and for program evaluation and reporting (Pool, 1996). Management and use of information generated by newborn hearing screening, evaluation, and intervention programs require careful consideration by service providers, state-specific lead coordinating agencies, statewide advisory committees, and state and federal funding and regulatory agencies. Federal and state agencies need to standardize data definitions to ensure the value of state registries and federal data sets and to prevent misleading or unreliable information (O'Neal, 1997). Information management should be used to improve services to infants and their families; to assess the quality of screening, evaluation, and intervention; and to facilitate collection of data on demographics of neonatal and infant hearing loss.

To achieve the first goal of improving services to infants and their families, multiple system components (e.g., hospitals, practitioners, public health, and public and private education agencies) that provide care for infants and families should be integrated. Optimally, and within the limits of confidentiality as defined by state regulation and parental informed consent, each service provider within the EHDI system (e.g., hospital, practitioner, public health agency, and public and private education agencies) participates in information management in order to track elements of care to each infant and family. The information obtained while using an effective information management system allows for the accurate and timely description of services provided to each infant and documents recommendations for follow-up and referral to other providers. Such information permits prospective monitoring of outcomes for each infant screened and assures that each infant is connected to the services he or she needs.

In addition to ensuring that each infant receives all needed services, effective information management is used to promote program measurement and accountability. Although recent survey data suggest that hospitals are successfully initiating universal screening, EHDI services including confirmation of hearing loss, fitting of amplification, and initiation of early intervention remain delayed (Arehart, Yoshinaga-Itano, Thomson, Gabbard, & Stredler Brown, 1998). One factor contributing to the delay beyond the 1994 and 2000 JCIH recommendations may be that few states have mandatory statewide information management, similar to that described here, that is capable of spanning the entire EHDI process (Hayes, 1999).

The information obtained from the information management system should assist both the individual provider and the lead coordinating agency in measuring quality indicators associated with program services (e.g., screening, evaluation, and/or intervention). Those professionals closest to the process should be responsible for program evaluation using the benchmarks and quality indicators suggested in this document. The information system should provide the measurement tools to determine the degree to which each process (e.g., screening, evaluation, and intervention) is stable, sustainable, and conforms to program benchmarks. Timely and accurate monitoring of relevant quality measures is essential.

Effective information management is capable of aggregating individual infant data from multiple EHDI service providers including hospitals, practitioners, public health agencies, and public and private education agencies. This information provides the basis for evaluating the effectiveness of the EHDI programs in meeting program goals of universal screening, prompt evaluation, and early and effective intervention. Tracking families through the systems of screening, evaluation, and intervention will permit quantification of the number of infants requiring and receiving services, and document the types of service during a specific period. Tracking improves the ability to identify infants who are lost to follow-up at any stage of the EHDI process. Until centralized statewide tracking, reporting, and coordination are mandatory, the transition of infants and families from screening to confirmation of hearing loss to intervention will continue to be problematic (Diefendorf & Finitzo, 1997).

The JCIH endorses the concept of a national database to permit documentation of the demographics of neonatal hearing loss, including prevalence and etiology across the United States. The development of a national database, in which aggregate state data reside, is achievable only with standardization of data elements and definitions (O'Neal, 1997). Standardized data management systems will ensure that appropriate data are collected and transmitted from statewide EHDI programs to the national data system. Data transmitted from the states to the federal level need not include individually identifiable patient or family information.

The request for information moves from the federal level to the state level and from the state to the hospitals and practitioners. Requirements from federal levels drive what data are collected and maintained at the state and hospital level. The flow of information should move from the hospital and practitioner to the state and federal levels through an integrated information system. Hospitals may collect and monitor data not required at the state level. Not all data collected as part of a universal newborn hearing screening program at the hospital or by the practitioner are needed at the state level, especially for the infant who passes the birth hearing screening with no risk indicators. Similarly, states may choose to collect data and monitor an expanded data set not required at the federal level. Information on the care status of an individual infant is not needed at the federal level.

The Bureau of Maternal and Child Health (MCHB) currently requires that each state report two data items: the number of live births and the number of newborns screened for hearing loss during the birth admission. The Centers for Disease Control and Prevention (CDC) are requesting that states submit 10 data items. CDC in conjunction with the Directors of Speech and Hearing Programs in State Health and Welfare Agencies (DSHPSHWA)began a pilot effort in 1999 to assess the feasibility and logistics of developing and reporting a national EHDI data set. The Pilot National Data Set includes the number of birthing hospitals in the state and the number of hospitals with universal hearing screening programs; the number of live births in the state and the number of infants screened for hearing loss before discharge from the hospital; the number of infants referred for audiologic evaluation before 1 month of age and the number with an audiologic evaluation before 3 months; the number of infants with permanent congenital hearing loss; the mean, median, and minimum age of diagnosis of hearing loss for infants identified in a newborn hearing screening program; and the number of infants with permanent hearing loss receiving intervention by 6 months. Such data could be used to examine prevalence of hearing loss by state or region, to support legislation for services to infants who are hard of hearing and deaf and their families, and to provide national benchmarks and quality indicators.

IV. Future Directions

New opportunities and challenges are presented by the current efforts directed at the early identification, assessment, and intervention for newborns and very young infants with hearing loss. Ultimately, the development of communication skills commensurate with cognitive abilities and cultural beliefs in the preferred modality of the family is the goal for all infants and children who are hard of hearing and deaf. Achievement of this goal will permit these children to avail themselves of all educational, social, and vocational opportunities in order to achieve full participation in society across the life span. To assure that such opportunities are available, universities should assume responsibility for special-track, interdisciplinary, professional education programs on early intervention for the child who is deaf or hard of hearing. Universities should also introduce training in family systems, the grieving process, cultural diversity, and Deaf culture.

Early identification efforts will be enhanced by the new technology designed specifically for the detection of hearing loss in the newborn period. The growing demand for screening programs will necessitate screening technology that is both rapid and highly reliable. Techniques or combinations of techniques will be required to identify the site of the hearing loss (conductive, cochlear, or neural). The development of middle ear reflectance measures may someday enable screening programs to determine accurately if middle ear dysfunction is contributing to the screening test outcome.

Because of newborn hearing screening, it will be possible to determine what proportion of early onset hearing losses are truly congenital versus those that occur postnatally. It will be possible to determine which types of hearing losses are stable as opposed to fluctuating and/or progressive. Intervention strategies could be tailored to the expected clinical course for each infant. Intervention will also be aimed at preventing the onset or delaying the progression of sensorineural hearing losses. Thus, objective techniques must be developed to assess the integrity and physiology of the inner ear.

Increasing reports of the deleterious effects of auditory neuropathy support the need for prospective studies in large birth populations to determine its prevalence and natural history (Gravel & Stapells, 1993; Kraus, Ozdamar, Stein, & Reed, 1984; Sininger, Hood, Starr, Berlin, & and Picton, 1995; Starr, Picton,

Sininger, Hood, & Berlin, 1996; Stein et al., 1996). Consensus development is needed concerning appropriate early intervention strategies for infants with auditory neuropathy. As more information on this disorder becomes available, hearing screening protocols may need to be revised in order to allow the detection of auditory neuropathy in newborns.

The JCIH anticipates that the earliest audiologic assessments, and subsequently the determination of appropriate interventions, will continue to rely on the use of physiologic measures. In particular, ABR air- and bone-conduction techniques could be used for rapid, reliable, and frequency-specific threshold assessment. The further development of these techniques for use with very young infants would be useful in the early comprehensive assessment process. Timely evaluation of hearing sensitivity will prevent delay in confirming the existence of a hearing loss and initiating appropriate audiologic, medical/surgical, and developmental intervention.

Amplification fitting will rely on pediatric prescriptive formulas individualized with real-ear measures and modifications (such as real-ear-to-coupler differences) to select and evaluate hearing aid fittings. Technological advances in digital and programmable hearing aids and alternative strategies such as frequency transposition hearing aids will facilitate more effective early intervention. The age of cochlear implantation for profoundly deaf children may be lowered proportionately with the earlier age of identification. Accurate selection and fitting of these devices in the infant or very young child will require reliance on objective (physiologic) assessment tools as well. These predictive measures, such as electrical ABR or electrical middle ear muscle reflexes obtained with stimulation delivered via the implant, must be validated in older children and adults to prepare for use in infants and prelinguistic children.

Health, social service, and education agencies associated with early intervention and Head Start programs should be prepared for a dramatic escalation in the need for family-centered infant intervention services. Because of the early identification and intervention programs, the JCIH anticipates that children who are hard of hearing and deaf who have received early identification and intervention will perform quite differently from their later-identified peers. As these children enter formal education, systems will need the flexibility to assess and respond to the abilities of these children appropriately.

With advances in human genetic research and the completion of the national Human Genome Project, thousands of genes associated with a variety of conditions will be discovered in the coming decade (Khoury, 1999). The identification of 11 genes for nonsyndromic deafness reported by the end of 1998 (Morton, 1999) provides the impetus for formulating strategies for population-based studies in the genetics of hearing loss. Although many different genes may be associated with nonsyndromic deafness, research indicates that a few of these genes may be responsible for a significant percentage of these cases. DFNB1, which is a gene responsible for recessive, nonsyndromic, sensorineural hearing loss, has been found to cause approximately 15% of all infant hearing loss (Cohn et al., 1999; Denoyelle, 1999). Currently, tests for the common mutations will detect 95% of DFNB1 in Caucasian families without consanguinity (Green et al., 1999). A positive test outcome for DFNB1 will eliminate the need for a CT scan, perchlorate washout, and tests for retinitis pigmentosa.

Studies in the genetics of hearing loss could facilitate diagnosis, including identification of risk indicators for progressive or delayed-onset hearing loss. Advanced knowledge regarding recessive genes responsible for nonsyndromic hearing loss could dramatically reduce the number of children whose hearing loss is classified as etiologically unknown. Increased sophistication in diagnosis may lead to new techniques for medical and/or surgical intervention. Otobiological research into hair cell regeneration and protection may yield intervention strategies that can be employed to protect the sensory mechanisms from damage by environmental factors, such as chemotherapeutic agents or high levels of noise or progressive forms of hearing loss.

The public health issues, as well as the ethical and policy implications, involved in this type of research must be addressed. The perspectives of individuals who are hard of hearing and deaf must play a significant role in developing policies regarding the appropriate use of genetic testing and counseling for families who carry genes associated with hearing loss (Brick, 1999). Privacy issues, including the potential impact of this knowledge on educational and vocational opportunities, together with insurability, must be thoroughly considered.

These efforts will be facilitated by the federal government's new goals in Healthy People 2010, which are as follows:

- To increase to 100 the proportion of newborns served by state-sponsored early hearing detection and intervention programs.
- To provide 100 of newborns access to screening.
- To provide follow-up audiologic and medical evaluations before 3 months for infants requiring care.
- To provide access to intervention before 6 months for infants who are hard of hearing and deaf.

We must assure quality in EHDI services through available benchmarks and standards for each stage of the EHDI process. Accountability for the outcomes of audiologic and medical evaluation and intervention services as well as the screening process itself must be documented. Outcomes and quality indicators obtained at the hospital, community, state, and national levels should permit the community to draw conclusions about the EHDI process, including its fiscal accountability (Carpenter, Bender, Nash, & Cornman, 1996). Such information requires that data collection be standardized, prospective, and ongoing for the next decades. The relatively few children who are hard of hearing and deaf and who have had the benefit of an effective EHDI system demonstrate gains in language not commonly reported. Only when language and literacy performance data are available for a generation of children with hearing loss who received the benefit of early detection and intervention will the true cost of EHDI be known. When outcomes for infants and their families are compared to the costs of these services, the community can judge the value of EHDI.

REFERENCES

Agency for Health Care Policy and Research. (1995). *Using clinical practice guidelines to evaluate quality of care* (Vol. 2, Methods, AHCPR Pub. No. 95–0046). Washington, DC: U.S. Department of Health and Human Services Public Health Service.

American Academy of Audiology. (1998). Draft: Use of support personnel for newborn hearing screening. *Audiology Today,* 21–23.

American Academy of Pediatrics. (1992). Ad hoc task force on definition of the medical home. *Pediatrics, 90,* 5 (RE9262).

American Academy of Pediatrics. (1993, November). The medical home statement addendum. *American Academy of Pediatrics News.*

American Academy of Pediatrics. (1999a). Privacy protection of health information: Patient rights and pediatrician responsibilities. *Pediatrics, 104,* 973–977.

American Academy of Pediatrics. (1999b). Newborn and infant hearing loss: Detection and Intervention. Task Force on Newborn and Infant Hearing. *Pediatrics, 103,* 527–530.

American Speech-Language-Hearing Association. (1989). Communication-based services for infants, toddlers, and their families. *Asha, 31,* 32–34, 94.

American Speech-Language-Hearing Association. (1991). The use of FM amplification instruments for infants and preschool children with hearing impairment. *Asha, 33,* (Suppl.5), 1–2.

American Speech-Language-Hearing Association. (1997). Guidelines for audiologic screening. Rockville, MD: ASHA.

American Speech-Language-Hearing Association, American Academy of Audiology, & Alexander Graham Bell Association for the Deaf. (1997). A Model Universal Newborn/Infant Hearing Screening, Tracking, and Intervention Bill. Rockville, MD: ASHA.

Arehart, K. H., Yoshinaga-Itano, C., Thomson, V., Gabbard, S. A., & Stredler Brown, A. (1998). State of the States: The status of universal newborn screening, assessment, and intervention systems in 16 States. *American Journal of Audiology, 7,* 101–114.

Baker-Hawkins, S., & Easterbrooks, S. (Eds.). (1994). *Deaf and hard of hearing students: Educational service delivery guidelines.* Alexandria, VA: National Association of State Directors of Special Education.

Bamford, J. M. (1998). Early intervention: what then? In F. H. Bess (Ed.), *Children with hearing impairment: Contemporary trends,* (pp. 353–370). Nashville, TN: The Vanderbilt Bill Wilkerson Center Press.

Berlin, C. I., Bordelon, J., St. John, P., Wilensky, D., Hurley, A., Kluka, E., & Hood, L. J. (1999). Reversing click polarity may uncover auditory neuropathy in infants. *Ear and Hearing, 19*(1), 37–47.

Bess, F. H. (1998). *Children with hearing impairment: Contemporary trends.* Nashville, TN: Vanderbilt Bill Wilkerson Center Press.

Bess, F. H., Dodd-Murphy, J., & Parker, R. A. (1998). Children with minimal sensorineural hearing loss: Prevalence, educational performance, and functional status. *Ear and Hearing, 19,* 339–354.

Bess, F. H., & McConnell, F. E. (1981). *Audiology education and the hearing impaired child.* St. Louis: C. V. Mosby Company.

Bess, F. H., & Tharpe, A. M. (1984). Unilateral hearing impairment in children. *Pediatrics, 74,* 206–216.

Bess, F. H., & Tharpe, A. M. (1986). An introduction to unilateral sensorineural hearing loss in children. *Ear and Hearing, 7*(1), 3–13.

Blair, J. C., Peterson, M. E., & Vieweg, S. H. (1985). The effects of mild sensorineural hearing loss on academic performance of young school-age children. *The Volta Review, 87*(2), 87–93.

Brick, K. (1999, June 7). *Genetics of deafness, deaf people and the past, present and future.* Workshop on the Genetics of Congenital Hearing Impairment. Centers for Disease Control and Prevention and Gallaudet University, Atlanta, GA.

Brookhouser, P., Worthington, D., & Kelly, W. (1994). Fluctuating and or progressive sensorineural hearing loss in children. *Laryngoscope, 104,* 958–964.

Calderon, R., Bargones, J., & Sidman, S. (1998). Characteristics of hearing families and their young deaf and hard of hearing children: Early intervention follow-up. *American Annals of the Deaf, 143,* 347–362.

Carney, A., and Moeller, M. P. (1998). Treatment efficacy: Hearing loss in children. *Journal of Speech and Hearing Research, 41,* S61-S84.

Carpenter, C., Bender, A. D., Nash, D. B., & Cornman, J. C. (1996). Must we choose between quality and cost containment? *Quality in Health Care, 5,* 223–229.

Centers for Disease Control and Prevention. (1997, November 14). Serious hearing impairment among children aged 3–10 years—Atlanta, GA, 1991–1993. *Morbidity and Mortality Weekly Report.*

Cherow, E., Dickman, D., & Epstein, S. (1999). Organization resources for families of children with deafness or hearing loss. In N. J. Roizen & A. O. Diefendorf (Eds.), *Pediatric Clinics of North America, 46,* 153–162.

Cherow, E., Matkin, N. D., & Trybus, R. (Eds.). (1985). *Hearing impaired children and youth with developmental disabilities: An interdisciplinary foundation for service.* Washington, DC: Gallaudet University Press.

Christensen, K. M., & Delgado, G. L. (1993). *Multicultural issues in deafness.* White Plains, NY: Longman Publishing Group.

Clark, T. (1993). SKI*HI: Applications for home-based intervention. In J. Roush and N. D. Matkin (Eds.), *Infants and toddlers with hearing loss: Family centered assessment and intervention* (pp. 237–251). Baltimore, MD: York Press, Inc.

Cohen, O. P. (1993). Educational needs of the African-American and Hispanic deaf children and youth. In K. M. Christensen & G. L. Delgado (Eds.), *Multicultural issues in deafness* (pp. 45–57). White Plains, NY: Longman Publishing Group.

Cohen, O. P. (1997). Giving all children a chance: Advantages of an anti-racist approach to education for deaf children. *American Annals of the Deaf, 142*(2), 80–82.

Cohen, O. P., Fischgrund, J., & Redding, R. (April, 1990). Deaf children from ethnic and racial minority backgrounds: An overview. *American Annals of the Deaf, 135,* 67–73.

Cohn, E., Kelley, P., Fowler, T., Gorga, M., Lefkowitz, D., Kuehn, H., Schaefer, G. B., Gobar, L., Hahn, F., Harris, D., & Kimberling, W. (1999). Clinical studies of families with hearing loss attributable to mutations in the connexin 26 gene (GJB2/DFNB1). *Pediatrics, 103,* 546–550.

Cone-Wesson, B., & Ramirez, G. M. (1997). Hearing sensitivity in newborns estimated from ABRs to bone-conducted sounds. *Journal of the American Academy of Audiology, 8,* 299–307.

Cone-Wesson, B., Vohr, B. R., Sininger, Y. S., Widen, J. E., Folsom, R. C., Gorga, M. P., & Norton, S. J. (in press). Identification of neonatal hearing impairment: Infants with hearing impairment. *Ear and Hearing.*

Corley, V., & Crabbe, L. (1999). Auditory neuropathy and a mitochondrial disorder in a child: A case study. *Journal of the American Academy of Audiology, 10,* 484–488.

Dalzell, L., Orlando, M., MacDonald, M., Berg, A., Bradley, M., Cacace, A., Campbell, D., DeCristofaro, J., Gravel, J., Greenberg, E., Gross, S., Pinheiro, J., Regan, J., Spivak, L., Stevens, F., & Prieve, B. (2000). The New York State universal newborn hearing screening demonstration project: Ages of hearing loss identification, hearing aid fitting and enrollment in early intervention. *Ear and Hearing, 21,* 118–130.

Davis, J., Elfenbein, J., Schum, R., & Bentler, R. (1986). Effects of mild and moderate hearing impairment on language, educational and psychosocial behavior of children. *Journal of Speech and Hearing Disorders, 51,* 53–62.

Davis, J., Shepard, N. T., Stelmachowicz, P. G., & Gorga, M. P. (1981). Characteristics of hearing-impaired children in the public schools: Pt. II—Psychoeducational data. *Journal of Speech and Hearing Disorders, 46,* 130–137.

Demmler, G. (1991). Infectious Diseases Society of America and Centers for Disease Control. Summary of a workshop on surveillance for congenital cytomegalovirus disease. *Review of Infectious Diseases, 13,* 315–329.

Denoyelle F., Marlin, S., Weil, D., Moatti, L., Chauvin, P., Garabedian, E. N., & Petit, C. (1999, April 17). Clinical features of the prevalent form of childhood deafness, DFNB1, due to a connexin-26 gene defect: Implications for genetic counseling. *Lancet, 353,* 1298–1303.

Diefendorf, A. O., & Finitzo, T. (1997). The state of the information. *American Journal of Audiology, 6,* 73.

Diefendorf, A. O., & Gravel, J. S. (1996). Behavioral observation and visual reinforcement audiometry. In S. Gerber (Ed.), *Handbook of pediatric audiology* (pp. 55–83). Washington, DC: Gallaudet University Press.

Doyle, K., Burggraaff, B., Fujikawa, S., Kim, J., & MacArthur, C. (1997). Neonatal hearing screening with otoscopy, auditory brainstem response and otoacoustic emissions. *Otolaryngology—Head and Neck Surgery, 116,* 597–603.

Eilers, R., Miskiel, E., Ozdamar, O., Urbano, R., & Widen, J. E. (1991). Optimization of automated hearing test algorithms: Simulations using an infant response model. *Ear and Hearing, 12,* 191–198.

Elssmann, S. A., Matkin, N. D., & Sabo, M. P. (1987, Sept.). Early identification of congenital sensorineural hearing impairment. *The Hearing Journal, 40*(9), 13–17.

Finitzo, T. (1999). The Sounds of Texas project: Principles from the 1994 Joint Committee on Infant Hearing Position Statement. In F. Grandori & M. Lutman, (Eds.), *The European Consensus Statement on Neonatal Hearing Screening* (pp. 38–43). Milan, Italy.

Finitzo, T., Albright, K., & O'Neal, J. (1998). The newborn with hearing loss: Detection in the nursery. *Pediatrics, 102,* 1452–1460.

Finitzo-Hieber, T., McCracken, G., & Brown, K. (1985). Prospective controlled evaluation of auditory function in neonates given netilmicin or amikacin. *Pediatrics, 106,* 129–135.

Fisher, R. M. (1994). The Mama Lere Home. In J. Roush & N. D. Matkin (Eds.), *Infants and toddlers with hearing loss: Family centered assessment and intervention* (pp. 195–213). Baltimore, MD: York Press, Inc.

Fletcher, R. H., Fletcher, S. W., & Wagner E. W. (1988). *Clinical epidemiology: The essentials.* (2nd ed.). Baltimore, MD: Williams & Wilkins.

Fortnum, H., & Davis, A. (1997). Epidemiology of permanent childhood hearing impairment in Trent Region, 1985–1993. *British Journal of Audiology, 31,* 409–446.

Friel-Patti, S., & Finitzo, T. (1990). Language learning in a prospective study of otitis media with effusion. *Journal of Speech Hearing Research, 33,* 188–194.

Friel-Patti, S., Finitzo, T., Meyerhoff, W., & Hieber, J. (1986). Speech-language learning and early middle ear disease: A procedural report. In J. Kavanaugh (Ed.), *Otitis media and child development* (pp. 129–138). Parkton, MD: York Press.

Friel-Patti, S., Finitzo-Hieber, T., Conti, G., & Brown, K. C. (1982). Language delay in infants associated with middle ear disease and mild, fluctuating hearing impairment. *Pediatric Infectious Diseases, 1*(2), 104–109.

Gallaudet University Center for Assessment and Demographic Study. (1998). Thirty years of the annual survey of deaf and hard of hearing children and youth: A glance over the decades. *American Annals of the Deaf, 142*(2), 72–76.

Glattke, T. J., Pafitis, I. A., Cummiskey, C., & Herer, G. R. (1995). Identification of hearing loss in children using measures of transient otoacoustic emission reproducibility. *American Journal of Audiology, 4(3),* 71–86.

Goldberg, D. M., & Flexer, C. (1993). Outcome survey of auditory-verbal graduates: Study of clinical efficacy. *Journal of the American Academy of Audiology, 4,* 189–200.

Gorga, M., Neely, S., Bergman, B., Beauchaine, K., Kaminski, J., Peters, J., & Jesteadt, W. (1993). Otoacoustic emissions from normal-hearing and hearing-impaired subjects: Distortion product responses. *Journal of the Acoustical Society of America, 93,* 2050–2060.

Gravel, J., Berg, A., Bradley, M., Cacace, A., Campbell, D., Dalzell, L., DeCristofaro, J., Greenberg, E., Gross, S., Orlando, M., Pinheiro, J., Regan, J., Spivak, L., Stevens, F., & Prieve, B. (2000). The New York State universal newborn hearing screening demonstration project: Effects of screening protocol on inpatient outcome measures. *Ear and Hearing, 21,* 131–140.

Gravel, J. S., & Hood, L. J. (1999). Pediatric audiologic assessment. In F. E. Musiek & W. F. Rintelmann (Eds.), *Contemporary perspectives in hearing assessment* (pp. 305–326). Boston: Allyn & Bacon.

Gravel, J. S., & Stapells, D. R. (1993). Behavioral, electrophysiologic, and otoacoustic measures from a child with auditory processing dysfunction: Case report. *Journal of the American Academy of Audiology, 4,* 412–419.

Gravel, J. S., & Wallace, I. F. (1992). Listening and language at 4 years of age: Effects of early otitis media. *Journal of Speech and Hearing Research, 35,* 588–595.

Green, G. E., Scott, D. A., McDonald, J. M., Woodworth, G. G., Sheffield, V. C., & Smith, R. J. (1999). Carrier rates in the Midwestern United States for GJB2 mutations causing inherited deafness. *Journal of the American Medical Association, 281,* 2211–2216.

Guralnick, M. J. (1997). Second generation research in the field of early intervention. In M. Guralnick (Ed.), *The effectiveness of early intervention* (pp. 3–20). Baltimore: Paul H. Brookes.

Harrison, M., & Roush, J. (1996). Age of suspicion, identification and intervention for infants and young children with hearing loss: A national study. *Ear and Hearing, 17,* 55–62.

Hayes, D. (1999). State programs for universal newborn hearing screening. In N. J. Roizen & A. O. Diefendorf (Eds.), *Pediatric Clinics of North America, 46,* 89–94.

Herrmann, B., Thornton, A., & Joseph, J. (1995). Automated infant screening using the ABR: Development and evaluation. *American Journal of Audiology, 4,* 6–14.

Hyde, M., Davidson, M. J., and Alberti, P. W. (1991). Auditory test strategy. In J. T. Jacobsen & J. L. Northern (Eds.), *Diagnostic audiology* (pp. 295–322). Austin, TX: Pro-Ed.

Hyde, M. L., Riko, K., & Malizia, K. (1990)., Audiometric accuracy of the click ABR in infants at risk for hearing loss. *Journal of the American Academy of Audiology, 1,* 59–66.

Hyde, M. L., Sininger, Y. S., & Don, M. (1998). Objective detection and analysis of ABR: An historical perspective. *Seminars in Hearing, 19,* 97–113.

Individuals with Disabilities Education Act Amendments of 1997. P. L. No. 105–17,111, Stat. 38 (1997). Codified as amended at 20 U. S. C. Section 1400–1485.

Infant Health and Development Program. (1990). Enhancing the outcomes of low-birth-weight, premature infants. *Journal of the American Medical Association, 263,* 3035–3042.

Jerger, J., & Hayes, D. (1976). The cross-check principal in pediatric audiology. *Archives of Otolaryngology, 102,* 614–620.

Jerger, S., Jerger, J., Alford, B. R, & Abrams, S. (1983). Development of speech intelligibility in children with recurrent otitis media. *Ear and Hearing, 4,* 138–145.

Johnson, D. (1999). *Deafness and vision disorders: Anatomy and physiology, assessment procedures, ocular anomalies and educational implications.* Springfield, IL: Charles Thomas, Publisher.

Joint Committee of the American Speech-Language-Hearing Association and the Council on Education of the Deaf. (1994, August). Service provision under the Individuals with Disabilities Education Act—Part H, as Amended, to children who are deaf and hard of hearing ages birth to 36 months. *Asha, 36,* 117–121.

Joint Committee on Infant Hearing. (1994a). Joint Committee on Infant Hearing 1994 Position Statement. *AAO-HNS Bulletin, 13,* 12.

Joint Committee on Infant Hearing. (1994b, December). Joint Committee on Infant Hearing. (1994). Position Statement. *Asha, 36,* 38–41.

Joint Committee on Infant Hearing. (1995a). Joint Committee on Infant Hearing 1994 Position Statement. *Audiology Today, 6,* 6–9.

Joint Committee on Infant Hearing. (1995b). Joint Committee on Infant Hearing 1994 Position Statement. *Pediatrics, 95,* 315.

Karchmer, M., & Allen, T. (1999). The functional assessment of deaf and hard of hearing students. *American Annals of the Deaf, 144,* 68–77.

Keefe, D. H., & Levi, E. (1996). Maturation of the middle ear and external ears: Acoustic power-based responses and reflectance tympanometry. *Ear and Hearing, 17,* 361–373.

Khoury, M. (1999). What happens after a gene is found? *Population research to use genetic information to improve health and prevent disease.* Presented at the Workshop on the Genetics of Congenital Hearing Impairment: Centers for Disease Control and Prevention and Gallaudet University, Atlanta, GA.

Kile, J. (1993). Identification of hearing impairment in children: A 25-year review. *The Transdisciplinary Journal, 3*(3), 155–164.

Kraus, N., Ozdamar, O., Stein, L., & Reed, N. (1984). Absent auditory brain stem response: Peripheral hearing loss or brain stem dysfunction? *Laryngoscope, 94,* 400–406.

Kuhl, P., Andruski, J., Chistovich, I., Chistovich, L., Kozhevnikova, E., Ryskina, V., Stolyarova, E., Sundberg, U., & Lacerda, F. (1997). Cross-language analysis of phonetic units in language addressed to infants. *Science, 277,* 684–686.

Kuhl, P. K., Williams, K. A., Lacerda, F., Stevens, K. N., & Lindblom, B. (1992). Linguistic experience alters phonetic perception in infants by 6 months of age. *Science, 255,* 606–608.

Littman, T., Demmler, G., Williams, S., Istas, A., & Griesser, C. (1995). Congenital asymptomatic cytomegalovirus infection and hearing loss. *Abstracts for the Association for Research in Otolaryngology, 19,* 40.

Luterman, D. (1985). The denial mechanism. *Ear and Hearing, 6*(1), 57–58.

Luterman, D., & Kurtzer-White, E. (1999). Identifying hearing loss: Parents' needs. *American Journal of Audiology, 8,* 8–13.

Mahshie, S. N. (1995). *Educating deaf children bilingually.* Washington, DC: Gallaudet University Press.

Marchant, C. D., McMillan, P. M., Shurin, P. A., Johnson, C. E., Turczyk, V. A., Feinstein, J. C., & Panek, D. M. (1986). Objective diagnosis of otitis media in early infancy by tympanometry and ipsilateral acoustic reflex thresholds. *Journal of Pediatrics, 109,* 590–595.

Marschark, M. (1997). *Raising and educating a deaf child.* New York: Oxford University Press.

Mason, J., & Hermann, K. R. (1998). Universal infant hearing screening by automated auditory brainstem response measurement. *Pediatrics, 101,* 221–228.

Matkin, N. D. (1988). Key considerations in counseling parents of hearing impaired children. *Seminars in Hearing,* 209–222.

McFarland, W., Simmons, F., & Jones, F. (1980). An automated hearing screening technique for newborns. *Journal of Speech and Hearing Disorders, 45,* 495.

Meadow-Orleans, K. P., Mertens, D. M., Sass-Lehrer, M., & Scott-Olson, K. (1997). Support services for parents and their children who are deaf or hard of hearing. *American Annals of the Deaf, 142,* 278–288.

Mehl, A. L., & Thomson, V. (1998). Newborn hearing screening: The great omission. *Pediatrics, 101,* e4.

Moeller, M. P. (2000, in press). Early intervention and language development in children who are deaf and hard of hearing. *Pediatrics.*

Moeller, M. P., & Condon, M. (1994). A collaborative, problem-solving approach to early intervention. In J. Roush & N. D. Matkin (Eds.), *Infants and toddlers with hearing loss: Identification, assessment and family-centered intervention* (pp. 163–192). Parkton, MD: York Press Inc.

Moses, K. (1985). Dynamic intervention with families. In E. Cherow, N. D. Matkin, & R. Trybus (Eds.), *Hearing impaired children and youth with developmental disabilities: An interdisciplinary foundation for service* (pp. 82–98). Washington, DC: Gallaudet University Press.

Morton, C. (1999, June 7). *The NIDCD Working Group on genetic testing for deafness and other communication disorders: Considerations for developing and implementing testing.* Presented at Workshop on the Genetics of Congenital Hearing Impairment: Centers for Disease Control and Prevention and Gallaudet University, Atlanta, GA.

National Institute on Deafness and other Communication Disorders. (1993, March 1–3). *National Institutes of Health Consensus Statement: Early identification of hearing impairment in infants and young children.* Bethesda, MD: Author. http://odp.od.nih.gov/consensus/cons/092/092

National Institute on Deafness and other Communication Disorders. (1997). *Recommendations of the NIDCD Working Group on Early Identification of Hearing Impairment on acceptable protocols for use in state-wide universal newborn hearing screening programs.* Bethesda, MD: NIDCD Clearing House (nidcd@aerie.com)

National Institute on Deafness and other Communication Disorders. (1998, Feb. 2–3). Economic and social realities of communication differences and disorders: Fact finding report. Bethesda, MD: Author.

National Institute on Deafness and Other Communication Disorders. (1999, September). *Communicating informed consent to individuals who are Deaf or hard-of-hearing* (DHHS, NIH Pub No. 00–4689). Bethesda, MD: Author.

Norton, S. J., Gorga, M. P. Widen, J. E., Folsom, R. C., Sininger, Y. S., Cone-Wesson, B., Vohr, B. R., & Fletcher, K. (in press). Identification of neonatal hearing impairment: A multi-center investigation. *Ear and Hearing.*

O'Donnell, N. S., & Galinsky, E. (1998). Measuring progress and results in early childhood system development. New York: Families and Work Institute. www.familiesandwork.org.

Ogden, P. (1996). *The silent garden.* Washington, DC: Gallaudet University Press.

O'Neal, J. (1997). From description to definition: Avoiding a tower of babel. *American Journal of Audiology, 6,* 73.

Oyler, R. F., Oyler, A. L., & Matkin, N. D. (1988). Unilateral hearing loss demographic and educational impact. *Language, Speech, and Hearing Services in Schools, 19,* 191–200.

Ozdamar, O., Delgado, R. E., Eilers, R. E., & Urbano R. C. (1994). Automated electrophysiologic hearing testing using a threshold-seeking algorithm. *Journal of the American Academy of Audiology, 5*(2), 77–88.

Ozdamar, O., Kraus, N., & Stein, L. (1983). Auditory brainstem responses in infants recovering from bacterial meningitis. *Archives of Otolaryngology—Head and Neck Surgery, 109,* 13–18.

Pediatric Working Group of the Conference on Amplification for Children with Auditory Deficits. (1996). Amplification for infants and children with hearing loss. *American Journal of Audiology, 5*(1), 53–68.

Pollack, D., Goldberg, D., & Coleffe-Schenck, N. (1997). *Educational audiology for the limited-hearing infant and preschooler: An auditory verbal program* (3rd ed.). Springfield, IL: Charles Thomas, Publisher.

Pool, K., & Finitzo, T. (1989). A computer-automated program for clinical assessment of the auditory brain stem response. *Ear and Hearing, 10,* 304–310.

Pool, K. D. (1996). Infant hearing detection programs: Accountability and information management. *Seminars in Hearing, 17,* 139–151.

Prieve, B., Gorga, M., Schmidt, A., Neely, S., Peters, J., Schulte, L., & Jesteadt, W. (1993). Analysis of transient-evoked otoacoustic emissions in normal-hearing and hearing-impaired ears. *Journal of the Acoustical Society of America, 93,* 3308–3319.

Prieve, B. A., Fitzgerald, T. S., Schulte, L. E., & Demp, D. T. (1997). Basic characteristics of distortion product otoacoustic emissions in infants and children. *Journal of the Acoustical Society of America, 102,* 2871–2879.

Prieve, B., Dalzell, L., Berg, A., Bradley, M., Cacace, A., Campbell, D., DeCristofaro, J., Gravel, J., Greenberg, E., Gross, S., Orlando, M., Pinheiro, J., Regan, J., Spivak, L., & Stevens, F. (2000). The New York State universal newborn hearing screening demonstration project: Outpatient outcome measures. *Ear and Hearing, 21,* 104–117.

Prieve, B., & Stevens, F. (2000). The New York State universal newborn hearing screening demonstration project: Introduction and overview. *Ear and Hearing, 21,* 85–91.

Psarommatis, I. M., Tsakanikos, M. D., Kontorgianni, A. D., Ntourniadakis, D. E., & Apostolopoulos, N. K. (1997). Profound hearing loss and presence of click-evoked otoacoustic emissions in the neonate: A report of two cases. *International Journal of Pediatric Otorhinolaryngology, 39,* 237–243.

Ramey C., & Ramey, S. L. (1992). Early intervention with disadvantaged children—To what effect? *Appl. Prev Psychol,* 1, 131–140.

Ramey, C., & Ramey, S. L. (1998). Prevention of intellectual disabilities: Early interventions to improve cognitive development. *Preventive Medicine, 27,* 224–232.

Rance, G., Beer, D. E., Cone-Wesson, B., Shepard, R. K., Dowell, R. C., King, A. M., Rickards, F. W., & Clark, G. M. (1999). Clinical findings for a group of infants and young children with auditory neuropathy. *Ear and Hearing, 20(3),* 238–252.

Rance, G., Rickards, F. W., Cohen, L. T., DeVidi, S., & Clark, G. M. (1995). The automated prediction of hearing thresholds in sleeping subjects using auditory steady state evoked potentials. *Ear and Hearing, 16,* 499–507.

Roberts, J. E., Burchinal, M. R., Medley, L. P., Zeisel, S. A., Mundy, M., Roush, J., Hooper, S., Bryant, D., & Henderson, F. W. (1995). Otitis media, hearing sensitivity, and maternal responsiveness in relation to language during infancy. *Journal of Pediatrics, 126,* 481–489.

Roizen, N. J. (1999). Etiology of hearing loss in children: Nongenetic causes. *Pediatric Clinics of North America,* 46(1), 49–64.

Ross, M. (1990). Implications of delay in detection and management of deafness. *Volta Review,* 92(2), 69–79.

Roush, J., & Matkin, N. D. (Eds.). (1994). *Infants and toddlers with hearing loss: Family-centered assessment and intervention.* Baltimore: York Press.

Rushmer, N. (1992). Parent-infant intervention strategies: A focus on relationships. In F. H. Bess & J. W. Hall III (Eds.). *Screening children for auditory function* (pp. 463–476). Nashville, TN: Bill Wilkerson Center Press.

Sackett, D. L., Haynes, R. B., & Tugwell, P. (1991). *Clinical epidemiology: A basic science for clinical medicine* (2nd ed.). Boston: Little, Brown and Company.

Schildroth, A. N., & Hotto, S. A. (1993). Annual survey of hearing-impaired children and youth: 1991–1992 school year. *American Annals of the Deaf, 138*(2), 163–171.

Schwartz, S. (1996). *Choices in deafness: A parent's guide to communication options* (2nd ed.). Bethesda, MD: Woodbine House.

Scott, D. M. (1998). Multicultural aspects of hearing disorders and audiology. In D. E. Battle (Ed.). *Communication disorders in multicultural populations* (2nd ed., pp. 335–354). Boston: Butterworth-Heinemann.

Sininger, Y. S., Abdala, C., & Cone-Wesson, B. (1997). Auditory threshold sensitivity of the human neonate as measured by the auditory brainstem response. *Hearing Research, 104,* 27–38.

Sininger, Y. S., Doyle, K. J., & Moore, J. K. (1999). The case for early identification of hearing loss in children. In N. J. Roizen & A. O. Diefendorf (Eds.). *Pediatric Clinics of North America,* 46, 1–13.

Sininger, Y. S., Hood, L. J., Starr, A., Berlin, C. I. and Picton, T. W. (1995). Hearing loss due to auditory neuropathy. *Audiology Today,* 7, 10–13.

Spivak, L. (1998). *Universal newborn hearing screening.* New York: Thieme.

Spivak, L., Dalzell, L., Berg, A., Bradley, M., Cacace, A., Campbell, D., DeCristofaro, J., Gravel, J., Greenberg, E., Gross, S., Orlando, M., Pinheiro, J., Regan, J., Stevens, F., & Prieve, B. (2000). The New York State universal newborn hearing screening demonstration project: Inpatient outcome measures. *Ear and Hearing, 21,* 92–103.

Stapells, D. R., Gravel, J. S., & Martin, B. A. (1995). Thresholds for auditory brainstem responses to tones in notched noise from infants and young children with normal hearing or sensorineural hearing loss. *Ear and Hearing, 16*(4), 361–371.

Starr, A., Picton, T. W., Sininger, Y., Hood, L. J., & Berlin, C. I. (1996). Auditory neuropathy. *Brain, 119,* 741–753.

Stein, L., Tremblay, K., Pasternak, J., Banerjee, S., Lindemann, K., & Kraus, N. (1996). Brainstem abnormalities in neonates with normal otoacoustic emissions. *Seminars in Hearing, 17,* 197–213.

Stelmachowicz, P. G. (1999). Hearing aid outcome measures for children. *Journal of the American Academy of Audiology, 10*(1), 14–25.

Stool, S. E., Berg, A. O., Berman, S., Carney, C. J., Cooley, J. R., Culpepper, L., Eavey R. D., Feagans, L. V., Finitzo, T., Friedman, E., et. al. (1994). *Managing otitis media with effusion in young children. Quick reference guide for clinicians* (AHCPR Publication 94–0623). Rockville, MD: Agency for Health Care Policy and Research, Public Health Service, U. S. Department of Health and Human Services.

Stredler-Brown, A. (1998). Early intervention for infants and toddlers who are deaf and hard of hearing: New perspectives. *Journal of Educational Audiology, 6,* 45–49.

Stredler-Brown, A., & Yoshinaga-Itano, C. (1994). Family assessment: A multidisciplinary evaluation tool. In J. Roush & N. D. Matkin (Eds.). *Infants and toddlers with hearing loss.* Baltimore, MD: York Press, Inc.

Tharpe, A. M., & Bess, F. H. (1999). Minimal, progressive, and fluctuating hearing losses in children: Characteristics, identification, and management. In N. J. Roizen and A. O. Diefendorf (Eds.), *Pediatric Clinics of North America, 46*(1), 65–78.

Tharpe, A. M., & Clayton, E. W. (1997). Newborn hearing screening: Issues in legal liability and quality assurance. *American Journal of Audiology, 6,* 5–12.

Thomblin, J. B., Spencer, L., Flock, S., Tyler, R., & Gantz, B. (1999). A comparison of language achievement in children with cochlear implants and children using hearing aids. *Journal of Speech, Language, and Hearing Research, 42,* 497–511.

Thompson, M. (1994). ECHI. In J. Roush & N. D. Matkin (Eds.). *Infants and toddlers with hearing loss: Family centered assessment and intervention* (pp. 253–275). Baltimore, MD: York Press, Inc.

Tomaski, S., & Grundfast, K. (1999). A stepwise approach to the diagnosis and treatment of hereditary hearing loss. In N. J. Roizen & A. O. Diefendorf (Eds.), *Pediatric Clinics of North America, 46*(1), 35–48.

U.S. Department of Education, Office of Special Education and Rehabilitative Services. (1998, Apr. 14). Final regula-tions: Early intervention program for infants and toddlers with disabilities. *Federal Register* (34 CFR Pt. 303).

U.S. Department of Health and Human Services. (2000). Healthy People 2010 (Conference ed., in Two Volumes). Washington, DC: January 2000

U.S. Department of Health and Human Services Public Health Service. (1990). *Healthy People 2000, National health promotion and disease prevention objectives for the nation* (DHHS Publication No. (PHS) 91–50212). Washington, DC: U.S. Government Printing Office.

Vohr, B. R., Carty, L., Moore P., & Letourneau, K. (1998). The Rhode Island Hearing Assessment Program: Experience with statewide hearing screening (1993–1996). *Journal of Pediatrics, 133,* 353–357.

Vohr, B. R., & Maxon, A. (1996). Screening infants for hearing impairment. *Journal of Pediatrics, 128,* 710–714.

Vohr, B. R., Widen, J. E., Cone-Wesson, B., Sininger, Y. S., Gorga, M. P., Folsom, R. C., & Norton, S. J. (in press). Identification of neonatal hearing impairment: Characteristics of infants in the neonatal intensive care unit (NICU) and well baby nursery. *Ear and Hearing.*

Wallace, I. F., Gravel, J. S., Ruben, R. J., McCarton, C. M., Stapells, D., & Bernstein, R. S. (1988). Otitis media, language outcome and auditory sensitivity. *Laryngoscope, 98,* 64–70.

Wheeler, D. J., & Chambers, D. S. (1986). *Understanding statistical process control.* Knoxville, TN: SPC Press, Inc.

White, K. R. & Maxon, A. B. (1999). Early identification of hearing loss: Implementing universal newborn hearing screening programs (MCHK125). Vienna, VA: National Maternal and Child Health Clearinghouse.\ Williamson, W. D., Demmler, G. J., Percy, A. K., & Catlin, F. I. (1992). Progressive hearing loss in infants with asymptomatic congenital cytomegalovirus infection. *Pediatrics, 90,* 862–866.

Yoshinaga-Itano, C. (1995). Efficacy of early identification and intervention. *Seminars in Hearing, 16,* 115–120.

Yoshinaga-Itano, C., Sedey, A., Coulter, D. K., & Mehl, A. L. (1998). Language of early and later identified children with hearing loss. *Pediatrics, 102,* 1161–1171.

* For reprints, contact Evelyn Cherow, American Speech-Language-Hearing Association.

Subject Index